KickStart to a Healthier You

Body, Soul & Spirit

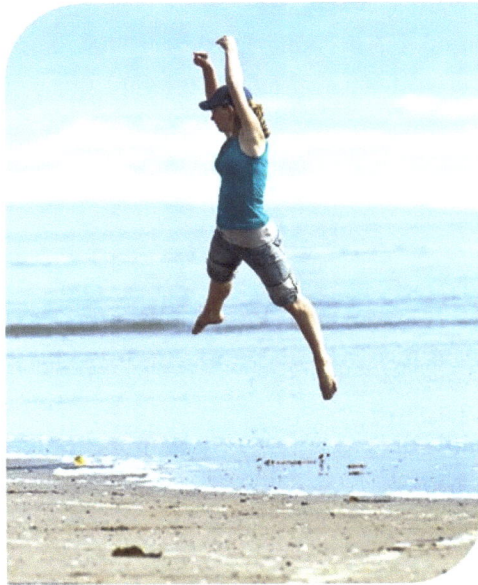

Dr. Carrie Wachsmann

Published by
HeartBeat Productions Inc.
Box 633, Abbotsford, BC, Canada V2T 6Z8
email: **info@heartbeat1.com**
604.852.3769

Interior photographs: Dr. Carrie Wachsmann
Cover image & page 2: Mike Baird   "A girl jumping on the beach."
Website: https://www.flickr.com/photos/72825507@N00/ Creative Commons
Editor: Dr. Win Wachsmann

Library and Archives Canada Cataloguing in Publication

Wachsmann, Carrie, 1952-, author

KickStart to a Healthier You – Body, Soul & Spirit/ Dr. Carrie Wachsmann
Includes index.

ISBN 978-1-895112-47-4

Printed in the USA

Using your Smartphone, and a QR reader app, take a picture of the code below and it will take you directly to my author's website at **carriewachsmann.com/blog**

Disclaimer

This e-book has been written to provide information about health and fitness and is for educational purposes only. Every effort has been made to make this eBook as complete and accurate as possible. However, there may be mistakes in typography or content. Also, this Book provides information only up to the publishing date. Therefore, this Book should be used as a guide - not as the ultimate source.

The purpose of this Book is to educate. The author and the publisher do not warrant that the information contained in this book is fully complete and shall not be responsible for any errors or omissions. The author and publisher shall have neither liability nor responsibility to any person or entity with respect to any loss or damage caused or alleged to be caused directly or indirectly by this book. (Kindle, eBook paperback, etc.) Check with your doctor before starting on any lifestyle changes that include diet and exercise.

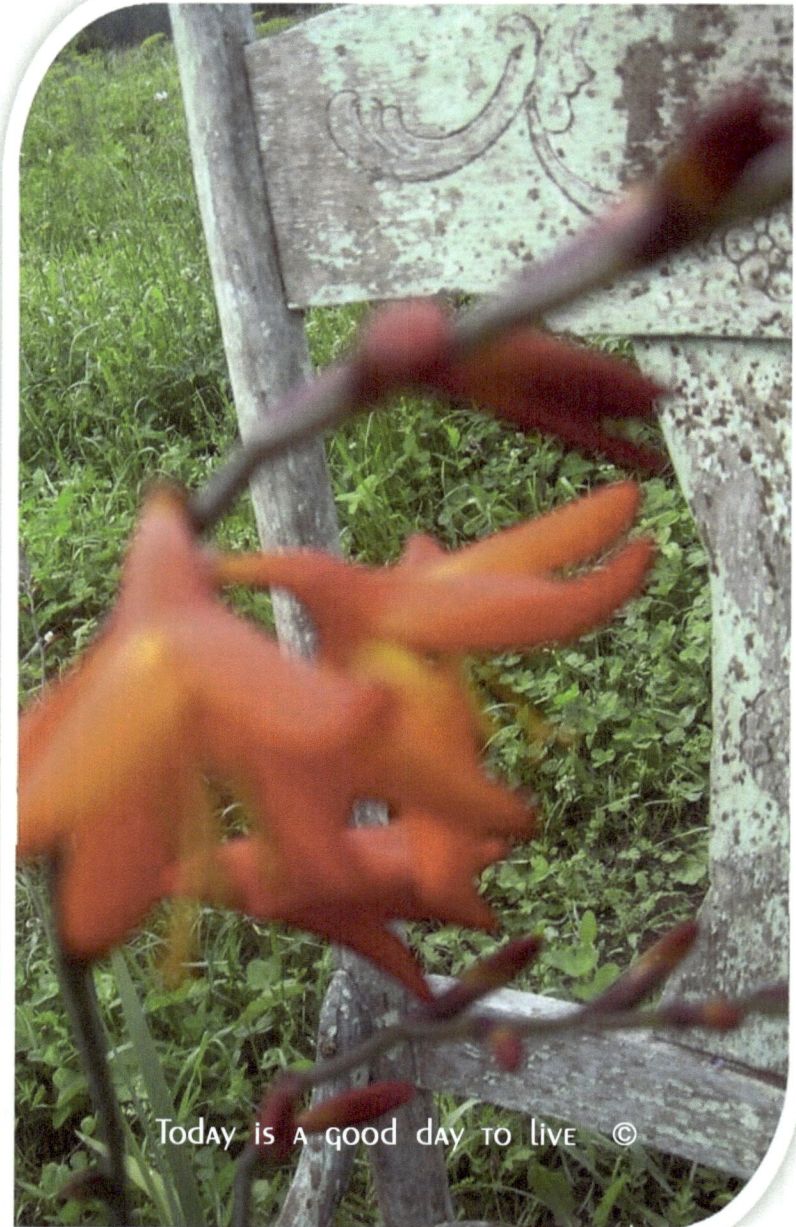

Today is a good day to live ©

Table of Contents

Tend the garden of
your soul

A garden does not need to be
perfect to be beautiful
and productive

Tend your soul garden well and
you will have plenty for your
family and others.
Neglect it and you will go Hungry ©

Chapter 1

Health Matters

You've decided to take charge of your health. You're serious and ready to put the time and effort it will take into creating a healthier you. Congratulations. You've taken the first important step in your journey.

It's no secret a healthy lifestyle is beneficial for everyone. Creating a positive mental state, making healthy food choices, and engaging in regular physical activities are all factors that contribute to your overall well-being.

When you maintain a balanced lifestyle, which includes a healthy body, mind (soul) and spirit, you'll be pleased to know the external stuff – all that stuff you can't control – will have little effect on your happiness and success in life. When you are in good health, your body looks better and is better able to ward off disease and disorders. The reality is you can create a better life if you are intentional about it, and this doesn't have anything to do with what is happening outside of you.

The holistic approach is the best way to take control of your health. This approach takes into account the complete person; your physical, psychological, social, and spiritual needs.

You can best improve your overall well-being by integrating all aspects of your being; not just by eating right and getting exercise. It's not just your physical body that needs addressing. Your mind needs stimulation; you need social interaction and long-term, healthy relationships. You need to nurture your spiritual side.

If you want to improve your overall health, you will have to make a long-term commitment to do whatever it takes to achieve that goal. You'll need to make lifestyle changes rather than just deciding to try a new diet for two weeks. Restricting foods or participating in a rigorous exercise regime for short periods of time will **not** produce the long-term benefits you desire. Although it seems to be a popular trend to try out the next new diet or be part of the next "exercise craze," these short bursts of diet and exercise changes don't provide lasting health benefits.

You will serve yourself much better by taking the time and effort to look at your whole self; preparing yourself mentally, gaining knowledge about healthy living, eliminating harmful habits, adding good habits, and discovering ways to nurture your inner self.

Your spiritual health is a vital component to a healthy and complete life. **Nurturing your body, mind, and spirit** is a package deal. You can't connect with your true self and commit to a renewed life of vibrant health without nourishing your spiritual side.

Chapter 2

Tend the Garden of your Soul

At one time or another in life's journey, everyone asks the question, "What is my purpose in life?" Discovering your purpose, discovering what motivates you and gives you the energy to continually grow, is part of your spiritual path. You were created as one-of-a-kind, with a unique set of gifts, talents and abilities wired right into your DNA. God spent some time thinking about you when He created you. It's up to you to develop those gifts, talents and abilities and to discover what significance your life plays in the world around you.

Your inner growth, your **soul garden**, is the most important growth, not only because it's what forms your perspective (which gives you a positive or negative take on your surroundings), but also because this is how you will discover the reason you were created. There's nothing more peaceful and satisfying than knowing that you're living your life the way you were designed to live it.

The **6 points** below will help you focus on living a life of purpose and meaning:

1. **Prepare the soil. Believe** you were created intentionally and have been given special qualities. Because God is on your side, with His help, you are capable of doing great and satisfying things. Take the time to talk to God about your concerns and ask Him for wisdom. After all, He created you and knows you best. Sometimes it's hard to know who God is and how He works in our lives. The best way to learn about God is to get to know the Jesus of the Bible, who told us "…if you see me, you have seen the Father (God)," John 14:9. Jesus is "The Way, The Truth and The Life, and no man comes to the Father (God) but through Him."

2. **Plant those seeds. Sow.** If you want to know more about this amazing Jesus of the Bible, read ***The Glorious Grace of God*** by *Lloanne Pinel*. This little book is filled with treasures straight from the Bible. Order here: ʜᴛᴛᴘs://ᴀᴍᴢɴ.ᴛᴏ/Ɜl4ᴀCCl

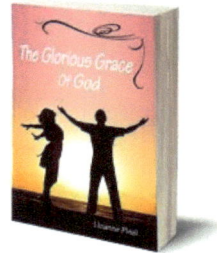

3. **Add water and sunshine. Be patient**—wait for the right things at the right time. Patience truely is a virtue. When you intentionally exercise patience, your ability to be patient will grow. Instant gratification is rampant in society today. Plant, water and hoe. Watch for it.

4. **Add some more water and sunshine. Generate love** continuously. To love under any circumstances is the greatest achievement of all. Practice it intentionally, and you will have success. Love helps to make the world work right. Love for yourself and others will make your inner world a much happier place. A loving God is our greatest example of how to love.

Dr. Caroline Leaf, author of *SWITCH ON MY BRAIN,* "...has researched the human brain with particular emphasis on unlocking its vast untapped potential. Her passion is to free people from their mental constraints and help them recognize their gift within."

Dr. Caroline says, people who view the world as being filled with love, are overall healthier, happier people.

5. **Pray over your garden. Weed it.** Develop a **practice of prayer**. Don't worry about all those rules out there about how to pray. You just need to have the intention to connect with your Creator with an honest heart. Tell Him what you're thankful for, what you'd like in your life and what you'd like for others. Ask him to help you change the things that need to be changed. Say it out loud, think it, and write it down in your very own prayer journal. Know that you have been heard.

6. **Appreciate your garden. Be aware of God's creation**. Nature is all around us, providing, nurturing, and sharing. Take time to spend quiet moments in natural surroundings and be aware of how perfectly nature lives. Take time to spend time in the great outdoors.

What about putting up a **birdhouse** or **bird feeder**?
If you are a novice, speak to your local bird store specialist to learn about bird feeders, to find out which birdhouse is best for which birds, which seed for which birds, etc.

You might consider planting a **small vegetable or flower garden**; either in boxes, in pots or in your backyard. Gardening can teach us much about tending the garden of the soul.

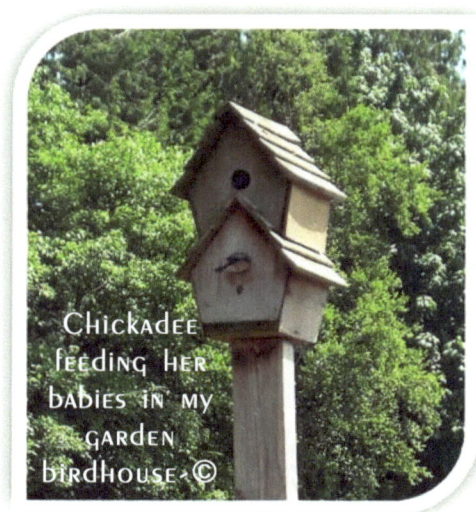

Chickadee feeding her babies in my garden birdhouse-©

No need to go big. With a little bit of love and care, a small garden can provide an abundance of produce and give plenty of rewards.

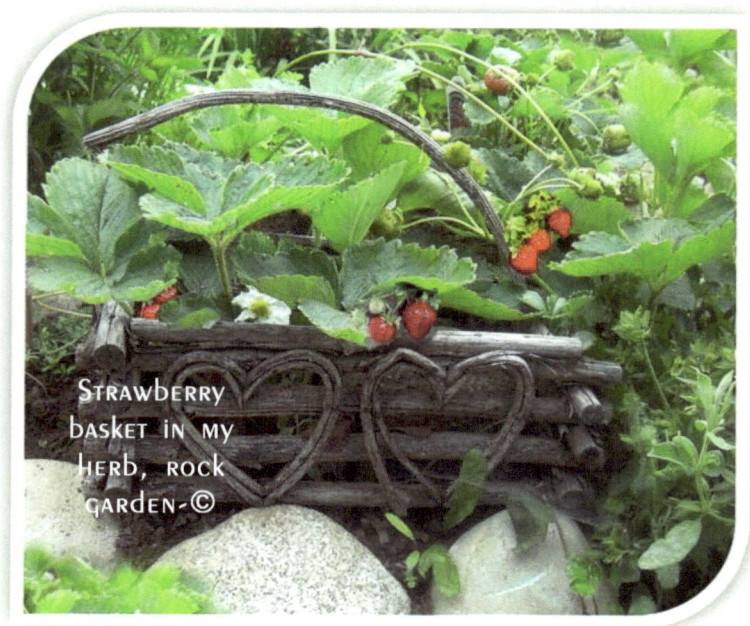

Strawberry basket in my herb, rock garden-©

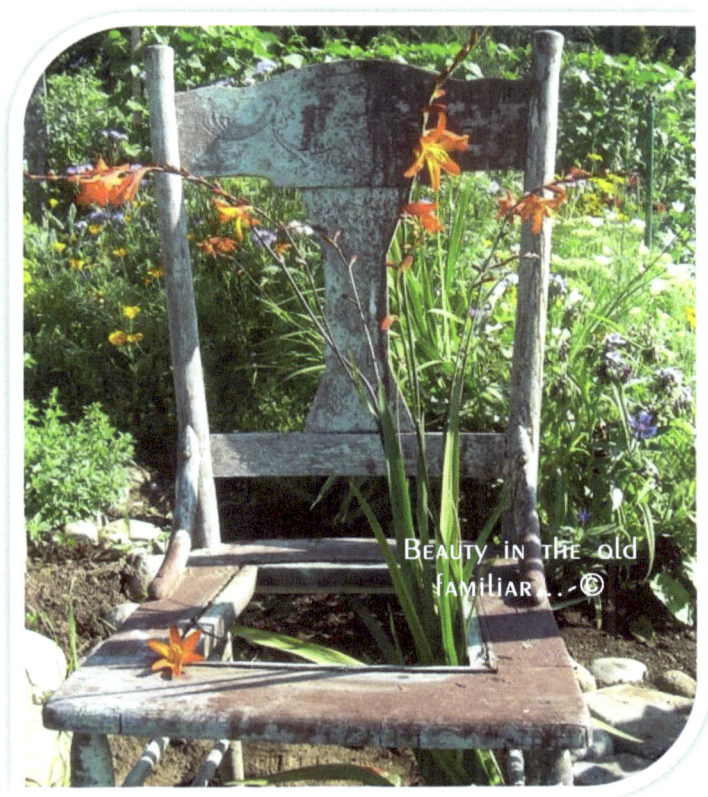

BEAUTY IN THE old familiar...©

Playing in the dirt is more satisfying and energizing than most people realize. Have some fun. It's not all about planting the seed, weeding and watering.

Let your creativity out of that box. This old chair was headed for the garbage!

You'll soon strengthen your faith in the God who gave you your unique set of gifts and abilities, and you can begin to live a truly blessed life. Planting a garden, watching it thrive as you weed, water and hoe is one of the best ways to grow your faith, patience, love, prayer life and belief in a loving Creator.

You were created for great things; things only you can accomplish, and it's up to you to act on those qualities with which you are blessed.

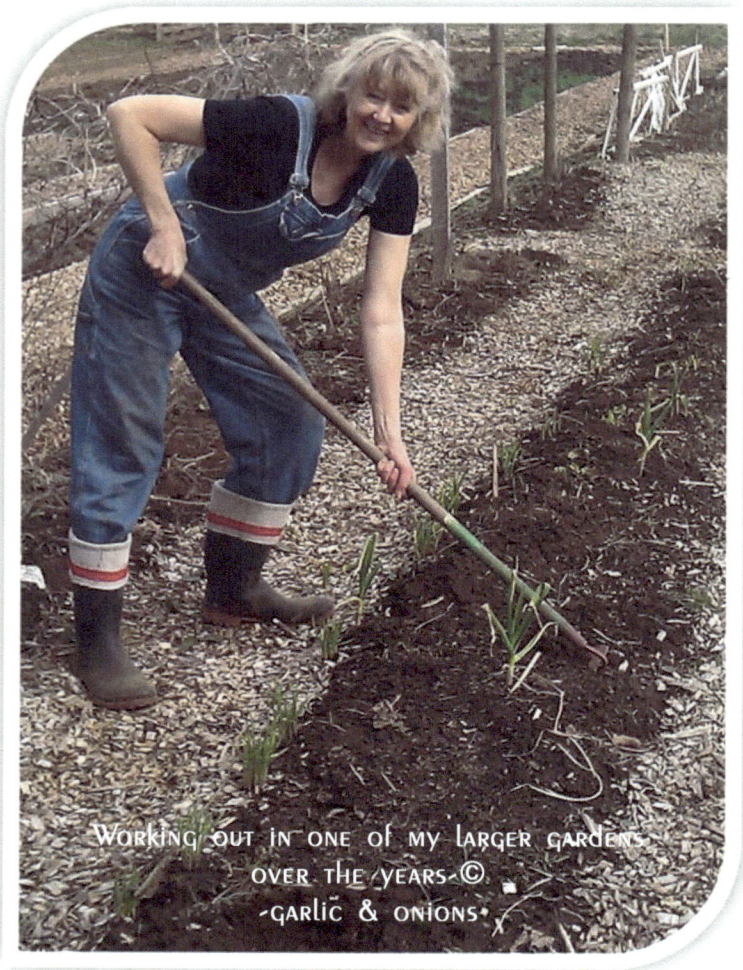

Working out in one of my larger gardens over the years.© -garlic & onions-

Living a happy life has little to do with what goes on around you, but rather a whole lot to do with how you perceive the world around you.

Chapter 3

Time to Begin Your Journey

You are strongly motivated to achieve a healthier you. You have a genuine belief in the reality of this healthier you. It's time to begin your journey.

Use the checklist below to help you set your goals and stay on track. Post it where you can see it daily. This checklist will help to keep you encouraged and strengthen your resolve.

You are sure to experience many benefits from a healthy lifestyle; some you may be aware of and some you will discover along the way.

What I can expect checklist:

1. A positive attitude about life and living
2. An open mind to experiencing new and nurturing activities
3. Less (or fewer) negative reactions and more control over your emotions
4. General benefits of physical activity such as increased energy, better muscle tone, improved metabolism and greater flexibility
5. Becoming more productive and effective in personal and professional activities

6. Experiencing a better quality of life
7. Reducing risk of chronic illness
8. Aspirations to achieve more in all areas of life
9. Reduced occurrence of bone loss associated with aging
10. Improving mood and self-esteem
11. Better functioning of all body systems
12. An overall sense of well-being
13. Looking forward to the future
14. A greater spiritual awareness

See page 18 for your "**Copy and Post**" list. This list is by no means complete. You will find yourself adding to this list over time.

As you can see, leading a healthy lifestyle is well worth the effort. Slowly but surely, you will be able to make the changes necessary for you to get the most out each day. As a result, your renewed optimism is sure to infect the people around you. So don't just make the lifestyle change for yourself. Do it for your children, your spouse, your parents, siblings, friends and even casual acquaintances. They will be inspired to take a closer look at their way of living when they see how full of life you are; all because you make your overall health a priority.

A few inspiring words to encourage you:

"A vigorous five-mile walk will do more good for an unhappy but otherwise healthy adult than all the medicine and psychology in the world." ~Paul Dudley White (1886-1973) American physician and cardiologist.

"Those who do not find time for exercise will have to find time for illness." ~Edward Smith-Stanley (1752-1834) English statesman and Prime Minister of the United Kingdom

"He who takes medicine and neglects his diet wastes the skill of his doctors." ~Chinese Proverb

"I pray that you prosper and be in good health, even as your soul prospers." ~3 John 1:2 - Christian Bible

Just because you're not sick doesn't mean you're healthy.

Never take good health for granted. Unfortunately, until it's in jeopardy, most people do not regard their health as a top priority. A sluggish body and a few extra pounds aren't a major cause for concern, but they are signs that there's room for improvement. Informing yourself by reading this book is an indication that you are aware health matters and you want to learn how to live healthier.

Perhaps you've already being working at improving your health or perhaps this is your first real introduction to a healthier way of life. Either way, this book will help you gain valuable knowledge and practical advice.

What I can expect Checklist:

Copy & Post

1. A positive attitude about life and living.
2. An open mind to experiencing new and nurturing activities.
3. Less (or fewer) negative reactions and more control over your emotions.
4. General benefits of physical activity such as increased energy, better muscle tone, improved metabolism and greater flexibility.
5. Becoming more productive and effective in personal and professional activities.
6. Experiencing a better quality of life.
7. Reducing risk of chronic illness.
8. Aspirations to achieve more in all areas of life.
9. Reduced occurrence of bone loss associated with aging.
10. Improving mood and self-esteem.
11. Better functioning of all body systems.
12. An overall sense of well-being.
13. Looking forward to the future.
14. A greater spiritual awareness and understanding of God's amazing love for you as an individual.

NOTES

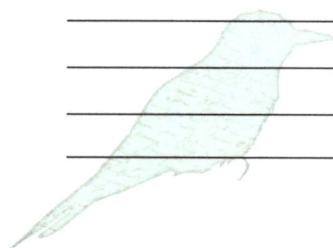

Chapter 4

Develop a Healthy Mindset

We are what we think!

As Caroline Leaf says in her book, *SWITCHED ON MY BRAIN,* *"Our bodies are a roadmap of our thoughts!"*

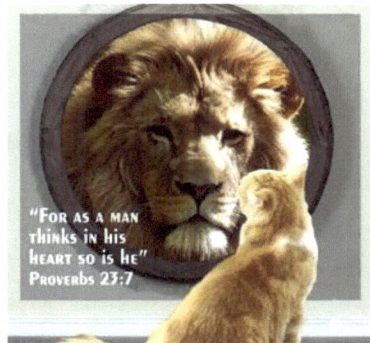

"FOR AS A MAN thinks in his heart so is he"
PROVERBS 23:7

A healthy mindset will help you in every area of your life; personal, relational, physical, spiritual.

FOR AS A MAN THINKS IN
HIS HEART, SO IS HE
PROVERBS 23:7

A healthy mindset understands that change is constant. Learning to work with change and embrace change is one aspect of a healthy mindset.

The question is—will you take control over that change?

Has anyone ever told you, "It's all in your head?" Interestingly enough, the battle is in our head—our minds—so if we want to get healthy, we better spend time getting our thoughts in line. Your thoughts can make or break your success in anything you aspire to achieve.

Knowledge is power

The first and most important step to getting in the **right mindset is** to arm yourself with **knowledge**. There is a wealth of information available on how and why to lead a healthier life, and you need to absorb as much as possible. There are several different methods for effective information gathering. Depending on your preferences, you will find some or all of the options on the following list helpful:

✔ **Search the internet** for any information about leading a healthier life. (Search *"healthy living tips" "making healthy changes")* Understanding the resistance to change (search *"breaking bad habits" "why it's hard to change"),* and connecting with others that are working towards a healthier lifestyle (search *"health forums," "health boards"*).

✔ **Study books** that will equip you with facts and tips for a health-focused lifestyle. The best type of book for this method is one you don't necessarily need to read from beginning to end, but you can read over time. Highlight sections and bookmark pages that are of special interest to you. Make the book your own by writing notes about your thoughts and experiences.

Examples—all favorites:

EATING ALIVE, PREVENTION THROUGH GOOD DIGESTION
HTTP://AMZN.TO/2Q8UU8X
- DR. JONN MATSEN

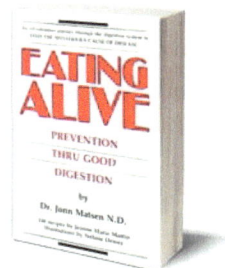

Switch on Your Brain -
Http://amzn.to/2oVilTS
- Dr. Caroline Leaf

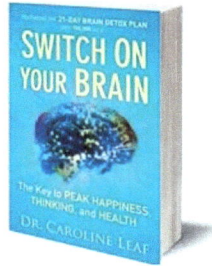

Foundations For Abundance -
Love, Joy, Peace, Patience,
Perserverance and Prosperity
https://amzn.to/32TnbBR
- Peter J. Dahl

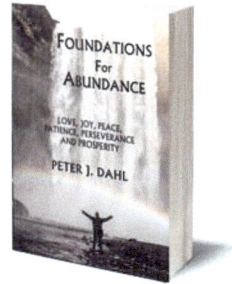

Magnificent Mind
at any Age
Http://amzn.to/2p2ymXQ
- Daniel G. Amen, M.D.

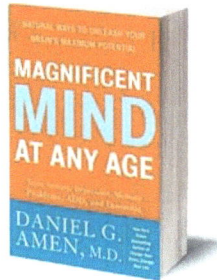

Live the Life you Love -
In Ten Step-By-Step Lessons
Https://amzn.to/2LIoaPS
- Barabara Sher

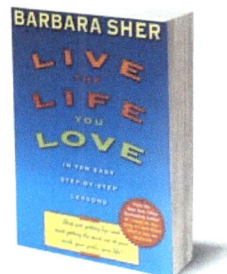

Living in God's Best
Http://amzn.to/2p4nZQs
- Andrew Wommack

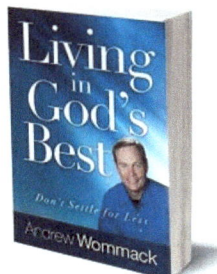

✔ **Record your thoughts** in your personal health journal or a blog. You may wish to Post your healthy living thoughts which allows you to connect with others on the topics. Connecting with others can also provide you with new insight and information about the many facets of healthy living.

✔ **Connect with people who are living healthier than you.** You are influenced by the people who surround you. Talking with, and spending time with well-balanced and happy people who are making healthy life choices, will influence you for good.

✔ **Get yourself an accountability partner** with whom you can check in regularly and share your health-focused journey. Although this could be someone who is already leading a healthy life as mentioned in the point above, **the accountability partner** is usually more effective if that person is someone who is in the same situation as you; someone who also needs an accountability partner—as long as that person is as committed to the process as you are. Look at this as a great opportunity for you to assist someone else and help them achieve **their** healthier lifestyle. By helping others, we naturally encourage and motivate ourselves.

✔ **Develop your self-awareness.** One area of self-awareness involves understanding pre-conceived notions you may have about food and your body. You may need to identify the underlying causes of unhealthy habits and find ways to **replace those harmful habits with good habits**. By taking this mental check-in before you make a lot of changes in your day-to-day activities, you can identify potential triggers and problem areas, which you will be able to address better when the time comes.

For instance, one of your unhealthy food habits may be eating regularly at fast-food restaurants; certainly not the best place to find wholesome food. You identify it's an easy source of food and, since you are not that great in the kitchen, you substitute fast-food for a well-balanced, home-cooked meal.

To address your well-established habit of fast-food eating you can educate yourself on the poor nutritional value and harmful ingredients often used in fast-food, and you can gain some knowledge about the value in the "slow food" way of eating. You can also learn how to make some quick and also healthy meals. **(See pages 64 - 88 for easy-to-make, healthy recipes**.)

✔ **Leave bad habits behind.** Most people say changing their habits is just too hard to do. Unfortunately, you can't avoid the hard part—the part where you have to deal with those well-ingrained, unhealthy habits. You can find comfort in knowing that anything worth doing is going to involve a struggle. Habits may take up to 21 days to change. The struggle and success go hand-in-hand. In the end, the struggle is worth it.

When we honestly analyze our actions and words, we will identify the bad habits that need to go in order to be able to function at our best. After that first step of deciding which bad habits we'd like to get rid of, we need to take action. Every one of us has a bad habit or two we need to deal with. So take up the challenge and don't let pride get in the way.

With persistence and determination, you can get rid of those useless and sometimes damaging habits for good.

> **Be intentional about your actions &
> stay focused on your desired outcome
> ...a life over which you have more control**

3 techniques to help you stop harmful habits

1. **Replace** those bad habits with good habits. For example, if you have a habit of talking negatively about other people, then make the decision every time you are tempted to talk or think badly about someone, then decide to think something good about them. Write down your intention on paper. Either post it somewhere you'll see it regularly throughout the day, or carry it around with you. You can find something good to say about pretty much everyone, even if it's just about their hairstyle or the color of their shoes. The point here is to shift your thinking from negative to positive, thus cultivating a much better mindset!

2. **Pick one habit** that you'd like to be rid of and focus on that one for a minimum of 21 days. The point of this technique is to exchange your bad habit for a good habit, and you can do this by spending a few minutes a day focusing on the desired outcome. In your "prayer" time, ask God to give you wisdom and insight into how best to overcome this habit.

3. **Use the power of writing things down** and write what you'd like to change. Follow up by making short notes every day about your progress.

You'll have days where you'll note you did the bad habit x number of times that day and you'll have days where you'll realize that you went through the whole day without giving in to the habit. Enlist your accountability partner. This person that you will be reporting to should not be judging your actions, but should merely be a listening ear and a source of encouragement. It's even more helpful if you were able to be their source of accountability as well.

Self-improvement takes time and patience. The worst thing you could do is overwhelm yourself with trying to change too much at once. The most common reason for failure to stop bad habits is not giving your goal or positive expected outcome daily attention. Don't make it lengthy or judgmental. Just be aware of what your intentions are and make a casual plan for change.

You also need to take action – not just think about change or just write down your ideas for change. We've all picked up bad habits, and its part of life to be be aware of what needs to go.

Know your stuff - strengthen your mind

Most people know what they want to stop doing and what they want to start doing but don't prepare themselves for the mental and emotional energy this change will take. Usually, they can maintain a week or two of working towards their ideal life, but without the mental preparation they slowly step back into their old routine, and before they know it, they've lost all motivation and progress is lost.
Has this happened to you?

The trick is to prepare your mind for the inevitable—at some point in this process, you will have the desire to revert to the old way. Make your new lifestyle aspirations a permanent shift, not just a temporary fad.

How can you do that? One way is to spend time researching and acquiring knowledge. You will want to determine your own personal potentially difficult-to-change areas and find ways to overcome those areas. I've experienced great success by trusting the God who loves me and created me, to help me be an overcomer. He is interested in our daily lives and wants to be part of it. Since He knows the end from the beginning, it's only wisdom to consult with Him daily

> **Be committed to your decision to be healthy; don't accept anything less**

In **Chapter 7** we'll talk more about how to foster a healthy mindset.

We'll end this chapter with an excerpt from **RICHARD CARLSON'S BOOK** - *YOU CAN FEEL GOOD AGAIN:* (also the author of - *DON'T SWEAT THE SMALL STUFF*)

> *"Commitment is a powerful tool for change. It takes pressure off of you by removing the uncertainty that often accompanies a lack of commitment. Marriage, for example, is a commitment. ... Prior to marriage, people often feel insecure about losing their partner, but the commitment relieves their anxiety and gives them the freedom to "let go" of their concerns; it fosters hope.*
>
> *Without commitment, success in any venture is difficult..."*

Chapter 5

Healthier Fuel:
Changing Your Diet

What you feed your body has an impact on your whole being; not just your physical self, but also your emotional, social, mental and spiritual self. How the body uses food affects every part of your being. Fuel your body with the most appropriate nutrients, avoid all unnecessary "filler" foods and you'll experience more benefits than just feeling great—you'll have a hard time avoiding physical activity.

You pretty much have to be living under a rock to avoid being regularly bombarded by advertisements regarding foods that are supposedly "healthy" for you. You need to get the facts from unbiased sources to be sure you're getting the most accurate information and advice about what is the right combination of nutrients and macronutrients (the protein, fat, and carbohydrates) that will supply the optimum performance fuel for your body.

Change the way you think about food

Changing the way you think about food will help you change your diet to a healthier one. Food is not only for your emotional pleasure, but a source of fuel to provide your body the needed energy to function properly.

NOTES

> ## Do you eat to live or do you live to eat?

Once you set your mind to healthy eating, (focusing on eating to live, rather than living to eat) you open your mind to exploring the many different foods - grains, fruits, vegetables you might otherwise never think to eat. Soon you will notice significant changes in your overall well-being. You'll begin to feel stronger and be more energetic. The rewards are many.

My son-in-law, who knows the intricacies of high-end, luxury vehicles says, "A high-performance car needs high-performance fuel which contains only essentials for the engine to function." In the same way, if your body were to run on high-performance food and not have to process food with little or no nutritional value, then you would soon find your body running smoothly and efficiently.

Changing eating habits isn't easy, so to make changes that stick, you'll want to use the following tidbits of advice to help develop your new way of fueling your body.

Tidbits of advice

✔ **Keep a record of the food you eat and what you drink—for at least a week**. This exercise will help you constructively judge your eating habits and identify areas for change, as well as make you accountable for your food choices. Studies show this to be one of the vital components to successful diet change and weight loss.

✔ **Eat slowly**, allowing your body time to signal when you're full. You'll also find, when you eat slowly you can appreciate the flavor of food more.

✔ **No need to count calories and measure portion sizes**. Be more concerned with making food choices that are in their most natural state (vegetable, fruits, grains, unprocessed meats and much more), and include color and variety.

✔ **Making small, but consistent changes over time** is a good way to achieve your goals for a healthier you. For example, if you want to consume more vegetables, start by preparing an array of raw vegetables to have on hand for snacking. Make this your goal for the week. Then the following week, you may want to start creating some dinner recipes focused on more healthy ingredients. Little by little you will be building new habits that will stick.

✔ **Drink water regularly throughout the day**. Water flushes toxins and waste products out of the body, which in turn helps you feel more energetic, gets you think more clearly, improves the appearance of your skin, and helps you to feel less hungry.

If you're not drinking around **2 liters of purified water a day,** you will want to implement this as one of your first life-style changes.

✔ **Moderation is the key** so don't feel like you can never enjoy your favorite sweet or the convenience of fast-food. Just don't make it a habit. Use moderation and balance with portion sizes. Don't fill your plate with a high-carb portion of pasta and only include a small serving of low-carb vegetables.

Although carbohydrates are an important part of a healthy diet, they sometimes make up too much of our diet.

Consuming too many carbs is not conducive to your body's optimum performance.

✔ **Try not to eat anything within 3 hours of going to sleep**. Studies suggest that this simple dietary change is beneficial for the digestive system. Especially avoid snacking on high-fat/high-calorie foods after the last meal of the day.

✔ **Learn to like the good sources of fat.** Fat tends to get a bad reputation for being the main contributor to weight gain, but it's mainly over-consumption of high carbohydrate foods that causes weight gain and a sluggish body. **Become well educated on the good sources of fat that are so vital to the nourishment of your body**. A couple of excellent options: nuts & seeds, olive oil, coconut oil, avocados, and fish.

✔ **Protein** is integral to building muscle and fuels the body with sustained energy. Eating protein (like eggs or isolate pea and brown rice protein powder in a smoothie) for breakfast is the best way to start your day. With toast and jam, you'll have quick energy, but it won't last long. A protein-packed breakfast will give you energy that lasts for hours.

Try not to put too much emphasis on **meat** protein. Some health consultants suggest limiting red meats and avoiding all processed meats. There is no need to completely eliminate meat from your diet, especially if you enjoy it.

Know what a **healthy portion is for your body, and eat the leanest cuts of unprocessed meat.**

✔ **Limit sugar and salt** and recognize all the hidden sources of these potential health threats. Although it's a given that consuming too much sugar and salt isn't ideal, the biggest thing is for you to be informed enough to realize all the places these ingredients hide.

For the most part, your food sources are going to start becoming more and more natural, but there will still be opportunities for the sugar and salt to sneak their way into your meals without you even realizing it. Keep in mind that salt is commonly used to cure meats and to preserve canned foods and commonly referred to as sodium chloride.

Alternate terms for sugar

The names listed below are names you will find on most ingredient labels. Be aware; these names refer to sugar.

1. Dextrose
2. Fructose
3. Fructose from corn
4. Glucose
5. Maltose
6. Sucrose
7. Maltodextrin (dextrin)
8. Brown rice syrup
9. Cane sugar
10. Corn sweetener
11. Corn syrup
12. Cane juice
13. Fruit juice concentrates
14. Barley malt
15. Caramel
16. Ethyl maltol

Our body needs a certain amount of sugar and salt for us to live and function well.

Healthy alternative sugars

1. Coconut sugar
2. Real Maple Syrup
3. Raw honey
4. Dates
5. Organic Blackstrap Molasses
6. Stevia (leaf powder or extract)

From my research, one of the best forms of salt comes from the sea. **Sea salt** has many benefits. It contains 60+ trace minerals, which help you stay hydrated, as well as trace elements that your body needs for proper adrenal, immune and thyroid function. It also contains digestive enzyme enhancers which help your body absorb nutrients from the food you eat. Why not replace the table salt in your salt shaker with **Celtic Sea brand salt.**

The serious solution to sinful snacking

The best way to fuel your body is to consume good nutrients throughout the day. When you snack, make it a healthy one. Many people, especially adults with busy schedules will either avoid snacking altogether or, out of convenience, snack on high-processed, high-sugar, and low-nutrient-content food. Some people may not know any better and not understand the major drawbacks that come with poor snacking habits.

The best solution to body-damaging snacking, in a nutshell, is to...

Prepare your snacks ahead of time! Follow these guidelines for energy-boosting, body-building and mood-enhancing snacks.

✔ Only buy packaged snacks **after looking at the ingredient list** and determining there are no added preservatives - **MSG, sugar, artificial flavors** or any long ingredient names that you can't pronounce or aren't familiar with. As a general rule, anything with more than 5 ingredients is not likely to be a great choice. (See page **39** for alternate names for MSG)

✔ **Larabar** brand nut and fruit bars make a great on-the-run healthy, energy snack. The ingredients are pure and simple; a variety of nuts, and fruits, and coconut, coca or dates. You can find them online or in many of your local grocery stores. **You can also make your own.**

✔ **Eat raw, fresh, organic produce whenever possible.** Consuming mostly organic is a good rule, but since price can be a factor for some, whenever possible, try to purchase the organic fruits and vegetables listed below; the ones that are most effected by pesticides.

Fruits & veggies most affected by pesticides

1. Apples
2. Bell Peppers (in some areas)
3. Blueberries
4. Celery
5. Cherries
6. Imported grapes
7. Kale
8. Nectarines
9. Peaches
10. Potatoes
11. Spinach
12. Strawberries

You can educate yourself on food additives and pesticides here: **Environmental Working Group**.

http://www.ewg.org/research/ewg-s-dirty-dozen-guide-food-additives

✔ **Get creative with your snacking.** Cook up some healthy recipes and separate into serving size, so they are ready to munch on at a moment's notice or grab on the way out the door.

✔ Are you a chip fanatic? **Resist the conventional potato chips that are deep-fried and high in salt**. You can make your own potato chips. Thinly slice one large potato. Let the slices soak in cold water for 20 minutes. Drain and pat dry. Season with a sprinkle of sea salt or other herbs and roast in the oven until lightly browned. You'll be pleased with how tasty and crunchy your homemade potato chips are!

✔ Try **roasting** other vegetables. Cut **carrots, beets** or yams into thin strips. Sprinkle with olive oil and herbs of your choice. Why not try roasting **brussel sprouts**, **green beans** or **colored pepper** slices?

✔ **Fancy up your fruits and vegetables with savory dips and tangy sauces.** This will provide lots of variety along with a treat for your sweet tooth. Make your own sauces so you can control what's in them. Almond butter is a tasty treat with various fruits and vegetables.

✔ **Keep a supply of natural raw nuts in your fridge or freezer at all times.** Don't worry about the fat content in nuts; it's the good fat your body soaks up and uses to your benefit. You should be more concerned about over-consuming high-carb foods like refined wheat products and too many potatoes and white rice. In contrast, nuts are packed with protein, antioxidants and the body-friendly fat: omega-3 fatty acids!

A note about wheat: **organic, sprouted wheat** flour is best if you wish to eat wheat products. Organic wheat, unlike regular North American wheat, is not subjected to sprays, like Roundup for example. Unfortunately, our North American wheat is no longer as nutritious and easy-to-digest as it was when our ancestors farmed the land. Many people find their health improves significantly by cutting out the wheat from their diet. (Or, if you are not wheat intolerant, replacing it with organic, sprouted wheat products.)

Snack mainly on fruits and vegetables. Many people find it difficult to consume the required amount of fruits and vegetables the body craves to function at its peak performance. The art of juicing is one way to ensure the body gets its daily required fresh vegetables and fruits.

The healthy art of juicing

Juicing, or extracting the juice from fruits and vegetables, has become a common practice in some health-minded households today. Some people juice daily, others on occasion. Whether you juice daily or ever-so-often, juicing has significant health benefits.

NOTE: One can find juicers in most grocery and department stores. If you want to explore juicing, but don't want to spend a lot of money on a juicer, check your local thrift stores. I found an almost new Braun brand juicer for $5.

Juicing is an optimum way to be sure to get a healthy dose of your recommended daily intake of fruits and vegetables. Although juicing doesn't provide the fiber that eating the whole food does, you are getting concentrated vitamins, minerals, enzymes and phytonutrients, which are absorbed directly into your system. **Don't cut out eating whole fruits and vegetables altogether**, as the fiber is also essential to good health.

One reason juicing is popular is because one can consume vegetables and fruits that aren't quite so enjoyable to eat. Juice those "undesirables" along with some of the more appealing vegetables and fruits, and you'll hardly even notice the spinach and kale among the apples and carrots.

Another reason juicing is popular - it is one way of giving you a high-nutrient drink, **custom made** to your liking.

If you're short on time, how about a glass of low-in-sodium **V8 type** juice? This vitamin-rich juice is made up of tomatoes, carrots, romaine lettuce, beets, parsley watercress, and spinach. You can learn more about the nutritional benefits of **V8** type juice here:

http://healthbenefitsofeating.com/drinks/10-health-benefits-v8/
Note: Read the label and watch for hidden names for MSG.
See page 39 for a list of hidden names for MSG.

A note of caution when it comes to juicing fruits: Fruit has sugar so limit your fruit intake. Too much sugar can elevate blood sugar levels. Some fruits have higher sugar content than others. Educate yourself on fruit and sugar content and how many servings of fruit per day is good for you. Here is a helpful site.

http://www.thehealthyeatingguide.com/sugar-content-of-fruit/

NOTE: If you are sick, have diabetes or some other malady, you may want to ask your doctor or naturopath to help you implement the best diet for your needs.

Raw is best - much of the time

If your digestive tract is healthy, eating raw vegetables is best much of the time. Although you can still feel good about adding some cooked vegetables to your meal, a cooked vegetable will have a lower amount of those vital and sensitive micronutrients. The main reason—heat destroys many of the enzymes.

For those of you who enjoy eating your vegetables cooked, some vegetables have different health benefits when cooked as compared to eaten raw, so don't overlook the value of cooked vegetables. **Lightly steaming your vegetables is one way to preserve most of the enzymes and nutrients.**

Dr. Jonn Matsen's (North Shore Naturopathic Clinic, Vancouver B.C.) advises to lightly steam vegetables during cold winter months (for those living in such areas) when the body digests and processes food differently than it does during warm weather. **This is especially good advice for those who have digestive concerns or are prone to colds and flu when cold weather sets in.** He has developed an *Eating Alive Program* which you can learn more about on his website.

http://www.northshorenaturopathicclinic.ca/

Dr. Matsen's book, *EATING ALIVE - PREVENTION THROUGH GOOD DIGESTION,* has many helpful suggestions and insights for persons dealing with digestive tract issues or health issues.

http://www.northshorenaturopathicclinic.ca/eating-alive-prevention-thru-good-digestion/

I have visited Dr. Matsen's clinic and studied his book thoroughly. His advice was foundational in helping me reach and maintain the long-term lifestyle goals I've set for myself.

Keep yourself informed so you can avoid diet blunders. By educating yourself about the best foods for a healthy body, you can save yourself the additional risk of developing a wide range of diseases and disorders. The more you know, the better life will go, and your body will be an excellent example of your acquired knowledge in action.

NOTE: About MSG - "***Glutamate acid*** *is bound up as part of the protein and only released as **free glutamate** when a healthy body makes it happen. In healthy bodies, glutamic acid is normal, necessary, and doesn't act like MSG in the body. Unfortunately, in unhealthy individuals, problems may arise...*" The glutamine found naturally in healthy foods such as homemade bone broth or bone broth powder - both from organic grass fed cows - should not be a problem for most people.

*"The problem develops when glutamine gets past the blood-brain barrier and is metabolized to glutamate. **In healthy individuals this does not happen willy nilly but is tightly controlled by the body.** Glutamine is supposed to convert as needed to either glutamate, which can excite neurons, or to GABA, which has a calming effect. Both are needed by the body and brain. The glutamine found naturally in healthy foods such as homemade bone broth should not be a problem, but all bets are off if MSG in the diet has led to glutamate build-up and brain damage due to excitotoxicity."*
–Dr. Kaayla Daniel, co-author of
Nourishing Broth: An Old-Fashioned Remedy for the Modern World
https://www.kitchenstewardship.com/msg-homemade-soup-meat/

To help with reading labels and make shopping for groceries less overwhelming, **copy this list below and put it into your wallet or handbag.**

Hidden names for MSG

The list below **always** contains MSG (**processed free glutamic acid**)

Glutamic Acid (E 620)	Glutamate (E 620)
Monosodium Glutamate (E 621)	Monopotassium Glutamate (E 622)
Calcium Glutamate (E 623)	Monoammonium Glutamate (E 624)
Magnesium Glutamate (E 625)	Natrium Glutamate
Yeast Extract	Anything "hydrolyzed"
Any "hydrolyzed protein"	Calcium Caseinate
Sodium Caseinate	Yeast Food
Yeast Nutrient	Autolyzed Yeast
Gelatin	Textured Protein
Soy Protein	Soy Protein Concentrate
Soy Protein Isolate	Whey Protein
Whey Protein Concentrate	Whey Protein Isolate
Anything "—-protein"	Vetsin
Ajinomoto	Natural flavors (often contains MSG)

To learn more about MSG, and **why** you want to avoid it, visit: http://lifespa.com/sneaky-names-for-msg-check-your-labels/#

Chapter 6

Building Fitness

Exercising doesn't have to be a high-cardio session or a sweat-filled weightlifting experience. Approaching your health from a fitness point of view means including activity; the more variety, the more likely it is you'll look forward to physical activity. To lay the foundation for an active life, let's go over the benefits of exercise and how it can improve several areas of your life.

✔ An obvious benefit of **being active is weight reduction or maintaining a healthy weight**. Moving burns calories, so you're sure to get that benefit no matter what your mobility or physical condition.

✔ Regular physical activity will help you **manage or greatly reduce the risk of contracting various health conditions and diseases**. A few examples of these disorders and diseases are type 2 diabetes, depression, heart disease, certain types of cancer, osteoporosis, stroke, and arthritis.

✔ Exercise is one of the best **antidotes for depression.** Exercise helps you to feel happier and more relaxed. Various brain chemicals (endorphins) released when you exercise will lift your spirit and give you a more positive outlook.

✔ Once you get into the habit of exercising regularly, **you will feel more energetic**. When you increase your heart rate on a daily basis, you'll have a long-term flow of energy.

✔ Have trouble sleeping? Exercise to the rescue! Regular activity living **promotes a quicker and deeper sleep** (when completed at least 4-5 hours before bedtime).

✔ Here's the marriage relationship booster: for some people, regular physical activity **promotes a happier sex life**. The energy boost will get you feeling in the mood, and all those feel-good hormones released during exercise (endorphins, dopamine, adrenaline, and serotonin) work synergistically to make you feel happy and confident, all of which relates to an increased libido.

✔ Of course, there's the **buff, toned body** and **greater range of motion** you'll enjoy.

Whenever possible, before he writes a prescription for medicine, our family doctor writes out a prescription for an exercise program - one tailored to the patient's needs (age, health condition, etc.). He says, "*Most of the time, exercise is all that it takes to help the body get back into balance.*" That's good advice.

Physical activity that fits you

Outside of the going-to-the-gym-routine and joining fitness classes, there are several other ways you can fit more exercise into your day. Incorporating just a couple of these exercising examples will not only help you reap the benefits of exercise, but also create a lifestyle full of fun, new experiences, and a deeper inner awareness.

Exercising in the great outdoors has the added benefit of soaking in the natural surroundings. There are many easy ways to incorporate cardiovascular activities into your program, with little or no equipment and you can start right away.

✔ **Running or walking** – a brisk walk can be just as beneficial as running so don't go for the high-impact option thinking it's the healthier way. Apart from needing shoes with good support, especially for running, these two activities are possible at any time, without any extra equipment. Also, try to create a longer walk for yourself by parking far away from your intended destination. Or go for a quick walk in the middle of the day – just for the health of it!

✔ **Biking** – A bike is a great investment, and you don't need to go top-quality. Any bike that you can ride will do. Choosing to ride your bike instead of driving your vehicle is a popular way to get some exercise while going about your daily activities. It's great for the environment too!

✔ **Skiing/snowboarding/snowshoeing** – for those who live in cold and snowy climates, you can benefit by taking up some activity that is dependent on snow. Exercising in the cold, crisp air helps to build your immune system and condition your body to resist winter colds and flu.

✔ **Stair climbing** – If you have a set of stairs in your home, be intentional about using them for exercising purposes. You can naturally add some extra physical activity to your day by choosing to take a flight of stairs instead of an elevator when you're out and about doing errands.

✔ **Jumping on a trampoline** – an exercise trampoline is a very small investment but provides an easy source of exercise. This is a simple way to add ten minutes here and ten minutes there of activity. You can jump with two feet or alternating feet, spin and jump, jump-kick and do lot more fun high-cardio activity, all without high-impact.

A word of caution to those who've suffered back injuries or have compressed discs. The trampoline may not be the best choice for you. Check with your doctor which exercises are best suited for you.

✔ **Skipping** – not just for children, skipping provides a low-cost, easy way to get an excellent cardio workout and which provides benefits such as calorie burning, improved coordination, strengthening of core muscles and enhanced bone density.

Along with cardio activity, you will want to incorporate some flexibility and strength training exercise to get the full healthy effects of a well-cared-for body.

✔ **Pilates** – You can attend classes with a Pilates instructor. If you want to exercise at home, get a video that you can follow along with or do your own sequence of positions after you get familiar with some of the moves. Pilates focuses on increasing flexibility and muscle tone. Start with simple moves. As your strength and flexibility improve, you can ease your way into more challenging moves.

✔ **Bodyweight Training** – this type of exercise uses the weight and movement of your body to tone and build strong muscles. Many different exercises are considered bodyweight training.

✔ **Weight Lifting** – done with free weights, this is similar to bodyweight training with the addition of even more possibilities for exercises and a greater ability to build stronger muscles. Having just a couple of different sized weights allows you to experience a wide range of weight-bearing exercises while not having to own a lot of equipment.

✔ **Flexibility Training** – also referred to as stretching. Stretching is a basic natural bodily function which feels great after sleep or sitting for long periods. It is also a key fitness principle to having a healthy body. By stretching your body, you are extending and lengthening your joints. This increases flexibility and results in better control of all your movements throughout the day. Pilates is considered a form of flexibility training.

✔ **Stretches** are very important in any exercise program. You can incorporate the basic calf stretch, hamstring stretch, shoulder stretch, etc. into your daily routine. The image below shows a stretching routine option to do <u>before</u> high-intensity cardio exercises or <u>after</u> any physical activity when the muscles are warm and more easily lengthened.

"According to the American Council on Exercise, stretching is an integral component of fitness and should be a part of any workout program. The act of stretching elongates muscles and increases the body's range of motion. Additionally, scientific research indicates that stretching encourages muscle growth." (See page 47 for stretch chart)
http://www.livestrong.com/article/262328-does-stretching-help-muscle-growth/

One of my fitness instructors teaches stretches can increase muscle mass up to 30%, if done correctly and consistently.

✔ **Russian Systema** —my chosen exercise program...

You can learn more about this fascinating program at this site: http://www.russianmartialart.com/whatis.php and
http://www.nationaltrainingcentre.com/wp/adults-2/#russiansystema

"...In Systema, the synergy of three components creates a **TRUE WARRIOR - Combat Skill, Strong Spirit,** and **Healthy Body**."

This program has no grading or belts. It is a unique journey for each person working to the best of their abilities.

I train at National Training Center located in Abbotsford, BC, where I have access to the wisdom and expertise of exceptional instructors. Perhaps someone offers this specialized training in your area.

When you commit to a consistent exercise program tailored to your body needs, you will not have a problem sticking to it.

You will be pleasantly surprised to see how easily you can get fit and feel great. By all means, increase your exercise time to what feels right for you! But keep in mind, it is best not to get obsessed with exercise – there is more to life, after all.

Basic stretch chart

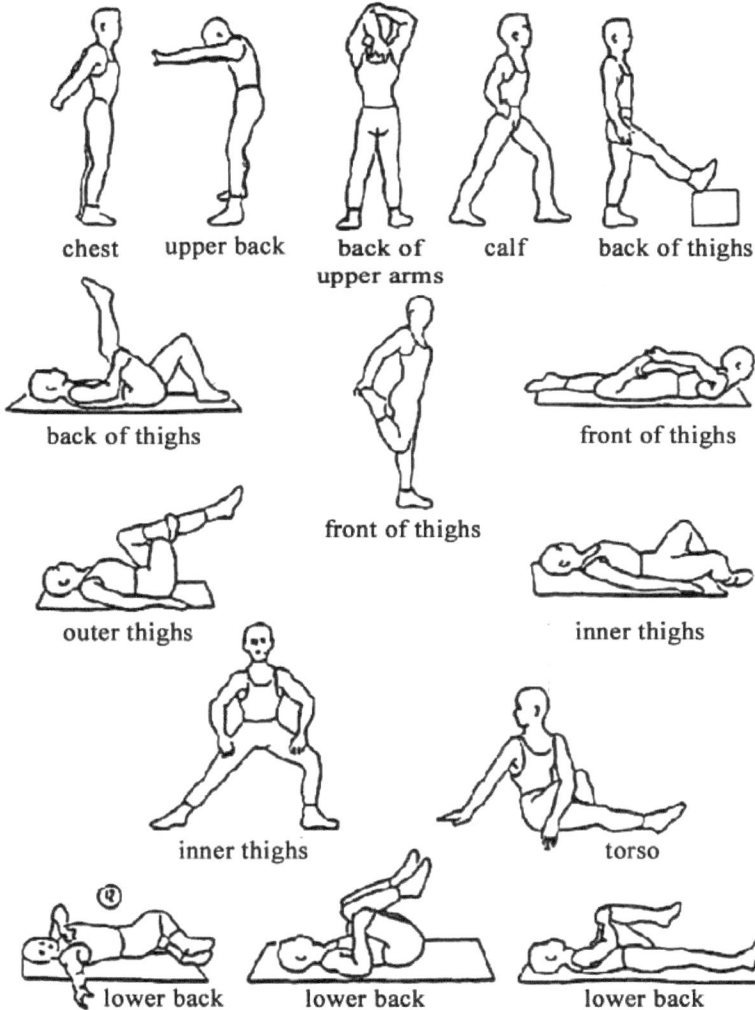

chest	upper back	back of upper arms	calf	back of thighs

back of thighs

front of thighs

front of thighs

outer thighs

inner thighs

inner thighs

torso

lower back

lower back

lower back

Get unstuck and experiment with different exercises. You should be doing what you enjoy in every area of your life. With the right attitude, you will have what it takes to handle life's challenges and "must do" tasks, and still enjoy your life.

NOTES

Chapter 7

Getting There:
Targets and Objectives

You're convinced taking care of your health is important. If you're going to commit to making significant, healthy changes in your life, you want to ensure you will be successful and maintain those changes.

You've got your journal and pen ready.

As discussed in Chapter 4, having the **right mindset** is essential and paramount to securing your success. A correct mindset will help you prepare for the emotional struggle that naturally comes with a lifestyle adjustment.

5 ways to establish a **right mindset** include:

1. Set milestones for achievement. Make sure they are achievable. The milestones you set will motivate you and help you reach your ultimate goal of an active and healthy life.

2. Put your milestones/goals on paper and post where you can see them daily.

3. Reward yourself when you successfully reach one of your milestones.

4. Talk. Talking about your goals and progress is the start to committing to the process.

5. Act. As the old saying goes, "talk is cheap" if not followed by **action**. You can talk about what you **want to do** and still fall short of your objectives. That's why it's so important to clarify your plan by putting it on paper. This creates a visual which will help you focus on your goals and help your subconscious to internalize your goals. That's what you want—depth and sincerity regarding your desires—not just "talk."

Do what it takes to keep the territory you've taken, and then confidently move on to the next milestone.

> **Create a plan, follow it through and gauge your progress along the way**

A very common system for setting goals uses the acronym

SMART as outlined below:

S pecific—Define your goals in a short direct statement.
M easureable—An example of a measurable goal is, "I will lose 10 pounds" as opposed to "I will lose weight."
A ttainable—Set goals you can achieve. Set plenty of morale-boosting smaller goals to help you work your way to the big one.
R ewarding—Make your goal an appealing reward. Something about which you can be excited.

T imebound—Set a time for completion. Don't agonize over an unreached goal in the predicted time. It's not a matter of completing a goal in the length of time set or don't do it at all. If the time comes and you still haven't attained your goal then just set a new date and adjust other components of the goal if needed.

Now, take some time to ask yourself these **6 questions:**
  1. Do I have bad habits I need to eliminate?
  2. Do I need to learn more about healthy nutrition?
  3. Who are my mentors?
  4. Am I aware of the exercises that are most effective for my body type?
  5. How will I keep myself accountable?
  6. What book/video will I read/study/watch first?

As you discover the answers to these questions, be sure to write them down in your progress journal.

Let's get practical by organizing your goals.
Organize your goals in a way that allows you to complete the simplest tasks first. Once completed, you can then move on to the more difficult tasks. Your successfully attained goals will motivate you.

In the military, a solder is expected to make his or her bed to perfection. Every morning at the break of dawn, this is the first task they tackle. Why is so much emphasis on excellence put into doing this seemingly mundane task? **Because it sets the stage for the rest of the day.** It sets the tone and attitude for the rest of the day. Your first job of the day was done with excellence and with a good attitude. Now, you are ready to take on whatever the day brings.

Look at the **sample set** of nutritional goals below to help you self-analysis your personal goals in the area of nutrition.

GOAL #1 - Spend some time going through ***Beautiful on Raw Uncooked Creations*** by Tonya Zavasta by February 25th.

Progress & Notes:

GOAL #2 - Prepare raw vegetables on Sundays and Wednesdays to use for juicing and snacking.

Progress & Notes: Be sure to record this every Sunday and Wednesday until you have at least 3 consecutive weeks of completing your goal.

GOAL #3 - Buy only natural (unprocessed) meats by May 2.

Progress & Notes:

Group your goals into:
> **Nutrition goals**
> **Fitness goals**
> **Emotional health goals**
> **Spiritual goals**

Write these goals in your health journal. Include a section for long-term goals you would like to achieve in 1-3 years.

I'm told, (I have not used this myself) you can find an excellent online resource to plan and track your goals at **http://trello.com**.
This site is designed as a project planner or task organizer and is very effective to plan and track goals.

There are several ways you can organize on this platform, so play around with it to work out the most effective process for you. This is useful for personal goal setting and implementation.

Another feature of Trello is the option to share certain boards or organizations with other Trello members. With this feature, you can add your accountability partner to your health goals board or organization, and they can check in on your progress and comment. Hopefully, you can connect with someone who is working towards some healthier living as well, and you can share your planning and progress.

Personal goal setting helps you to decide and choose what you want to achieve in life. You can use this same process of setting and implementing goals for any area of your life. Thinking about your ideal future and planning out the steps to get there is a powerful method that will in time, provide you with a great deal of personal satisfaction and fulfillment. This method also helps you realize more about yourself and your abilities, which in turn helps you to make the most of your life.

NOTES

GOAL #1 -

Progress & Notes:

GOAL #2 -

Progress & Notes:

GOAL #3 -

Progress & Notes:

Chapter 8

Setting a Healthy Example

When you've taken all the right steps to help you change your body for the better, you'll be able to calmly and confidently deal with the to-be-expected hurdles and setbacks. When you have a well-thought-out plan and a well-organized agenda, you can enjoy the process. All your efforts and enthusiasm will pay off, and you will have a positive effect on everyone you come in contact with. You will influence loved ones, acquaintances, and casual contacts by your dedication and commitment to taking care of yourself.

As you establish your success in the area of healthy living, you will be able to offer guidance and compassion to others who want to better themselves. Aspiring to be a good role model for those special people in your life can be motivation enough to stick with the "battle of change." While you'll start with questions, possible frustrations and uncertainty, you can feel confident that will soon pass.

You too can become a leader in the area of healthy living. Spread the happiness of healthy living.

"NEVER UNDERESTIMATE THE POWER OF A SMALL GROUP OF COMMITTED PEOPLE TO CHANGE THE WORLD. IN FACT, IT IS THE ONLY THING THAT EVER HAS." ~MARGARET MEAD

Because of your choice to be healthier, you have the opportunity to be an example to many people.

At one time in history, people could only source "natural" foods as found in their organic state. The hunter-gatherer diet of the past was plant-based with the addition of a meat product now and again. The body functions best when it's not overwhelmed with foreign or toxic substances it's forced to process. Today, we have to be intentional about what foods grace our table. We are overwhelmed with processed food options; refined and filled with additives. The body is put under constant strain when having to deal with "unnatural" substances found in our food, water and environment. Eventually, under the stress of having to process toxic substances constantly, our bodies can become susceptible to disease, discomfort, mental instability and other physical impairments.

You will inspire others

Change can be hard, but change for the better is rewarding. At this point, it's about you feeling good and getting your body in better shape. Your internal drive, planning and learning about a more natural way to live will keep you on track. When you achieve some of your goals, your new-found healthy perspective will subconsciously impress others.

Be prepared to be admired

Be prepared to be a mentor and be asked for your input. You may be a humble soul and assume your desire to be a better person isn't that big of a deal for other people, but it is!. Most likely, your immediate family will be affected, if only because they undoubtedly will be privy to your efforts.

Perhaps you were inspired by someone you knew who was taking control of their life and creating a healthier and happier lifestyle? You can be that person and be a positive role model for any number of people in your circle of friends and family. This thought should help you never give up on the health-focused life.

What if I'm a senior?

If you are a senior think about the impact you can have as you set the bar with your friends and family by aging gracefully. It's never too late, and you are never too old to make significant health changes.

If you need encouragement and a healthy "kick start," read about these elderly athletes who are "redefining old age."

http://www.telegraph.co.uk/lifestyle/wellbeing/11807078/The-elderly-athletes-redfining-old-age.html

http://www.aplaceformom.com/blog/5-amazing-elderly-athletes/

How about these 100-year-old teachers who keep on teaching?

http://www.huffingtonpost.com/news/100-year-old-teacher/

What's your excuse?

The world needs better role models, and you can become one of them.

If you're not quite up to the task of encouraging a healthy life for others at this point, that's OK. Take your time and get some success under your belt. I guarantee you'll feel up to it after you experience a few successes and you're well established in new healthy life!

"The world is a dangerous place to live; not because of the people who are evil, but because of the people who don't do anything about it." ~Albert Einstein

NOTES

_____

_____

_____

_____

_____

_____

_____

_____

_____

_____

_____

_____

_____

_____

Chapter 9

Are you up to the task?

If you've read this far, you are most likely "up to the task." You are ready to make some significant changes in your life. Your decision to be a healthier you is one of the most important decisions you'll make for yourself. Taking on healthier habits will open the door to achieving your true potential. You will not be held back by poor health and all the negative side-effects that come with it. As you probably know, you don't have to be diagnosed with a debilitating disease to have poor health affect you. Difficult to control emotions, lack of energy, disinterest in being active (which is contrary to the natural human condition to be striving, achieving and creating), and a myriad of other symptoms that can make life difficult, can affect you.

Some profound words from Isaac Asimov (1920-1992 American author and professor of biochemistry):

"It has been my philosophy of life that difficulties vanish when faced boldly."

Life can be a struggle, and we accept that. Be bold. One thing I've heard many people say when going through a difficult time, "…at least I've got my health."

Life seems to be so much more difficult when you have to face challenges involving your health on top of other difficult "stuff." If you already have health issues, you know what I'm talking about.

In the words of Hippocrates...
"Let food be thy medicine and medicine be thy food."

Words from long ago still speak true today. Eating the right foods and avoiding harmful foods will allow your body to heal itself.

Once you've equipped yourself with knowledge and sound advice to help take you through this process of change involving health, you may soon find other areas of your life you want to change.

Don't stop now -
become the person you want to be

As we talked about earlier, it's easy to say you want to change, but it takes persistence and motivation to act and make change happen. You are a product of your upbringing, and it's not always good stuff that surrounded you. As children, we are highly impressionable. We take those attitudes and perspectives we adopt as children with us into adulthood.

Even as adults, we're still susceptible to picking up bad habits and listening to the advice of perhaps well-meaning, but misguided individuals.

Decide what other things aren't working for you. **Focus** more on **how you want to be** instead of trying to figure out how you're going to stop being a certain way.

A few simple questions will help you define what is important for you and what areas of your life you need to strengthen.

1. What are your priorities concerning career, family, social activities, personal growth and spiritual growth?
2. What character traits do you admire in others? And you would like to have yourself?
3. Who do you know that is encouraging to be around? How do they add value to your life?

Write down your priorities, the character traits you want to develop, and the people with whom you should surround yourself. The answers to these questions will help you determine what other things you need to work on to make progress on your path to complete personal growth

To make those changes and be that better and wiser person, you need to dedicate some time to this process daily.

> **Imagine your life the way you want it to be**

Make an appointment with yourself each day to spend a few minutes imagining your life the way you want it to be. Jot thoughts down in your health journal, share them with your accountability partner and bring them up in conversation with others whose input your value.

Since personal growth in every area of your life is a lifelong endeavor, don't get overwhelmed and think you have to deal with everything at once. The steps you take to becoming a better healthier you are significant to your lifelong quest for purpose, health and happiness.

You never have to accept anything about yourself that you are not happy with, and with God on your side, you have the power to make that change happen—even if it's something that's been ingrained in you for years.

Stick to your plan, break free & take action!

You're making a decision to be free!
- ✔ To be free of unhealthy information
- ✔ To be free of constricting thoughts
- ✔ To be free of limited nutrition
- ✔ To be free of inactivity
- ✔ To be free of purposeless days
- ✔ To be free of an uninspiring life
- ✔ To be free of ignorance when it comes to your health
- ✔ To be free of wrong thinking in all areas of your life
- ✔ To be free to pursue your God-given destiny

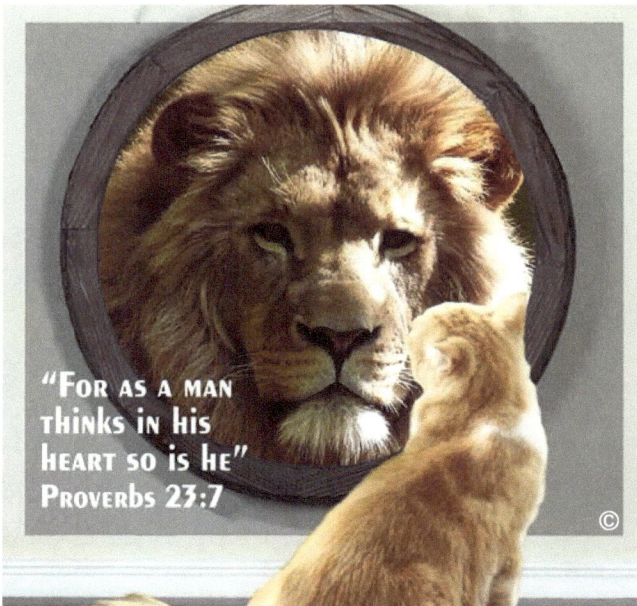

"FOR AS A MAN thinks in his heart so is he" Proverbs 23:7

Recommended Resources

👍 *EATING ALIVE - PREVENTION THROUGH GOOD DIGESTION*
DR. JOHN MATSEN
HTTP://AMZN.TO/2Q8UU8X

👍 *SWITCH ON YOUR BRAIN*
DR. CAROLINE LEAF
HTTP://AMZN.TO/2OVILTS

👍 *MAGNIFICENT MIND AT ANY AGE*
DANIEL G. AMEN, M.D.
HTTP://AMZN.TO/2P2YMXQ

👍 *FOUNDATIONS FOR ABUNDANCE - LOVE, JOY, PEACE, PATIENCE, PERSEVERANCE AND PROSPERITY*
PETER J. DAHL
HTTPS://AMZN.TO/32TNBBR

👍 *LIVE THE LIFE YOU LOVE - IN TEN STEP-BY-STEP LESSONS*
BARABARA SHER
HTTPS://AMZN.TO/2LIOAPS

👍 *THE GLORIOUS GRACE OF GOD*
LLOANNE PINEL
HTTPS://AMZN.TO/314ACCL

👍 *LIVING IN GOD'S BEST*
ANDREW WOMMACK
HTTP://AMZN.TO/2P4NJAY

👍 *BEAUTIFUL ON RAW UNCOOKED CREATIONS*
(NOTE: JUICING RECIPES & EDUCATION ON RAW foods)
TONYA ZAVASTA
HTTP://AMZN.TO/2QJKOTP

👍 *HEALTHY RECIPES* - Food is Medicine Website
DR. AXE
HTTPS://DRAXE.COM/SECTION/RECIPES/#RESULTS

NOTES

Sampling of Carrie's Tried & True Healthy Recipes

1. No Guilt Energy Bar

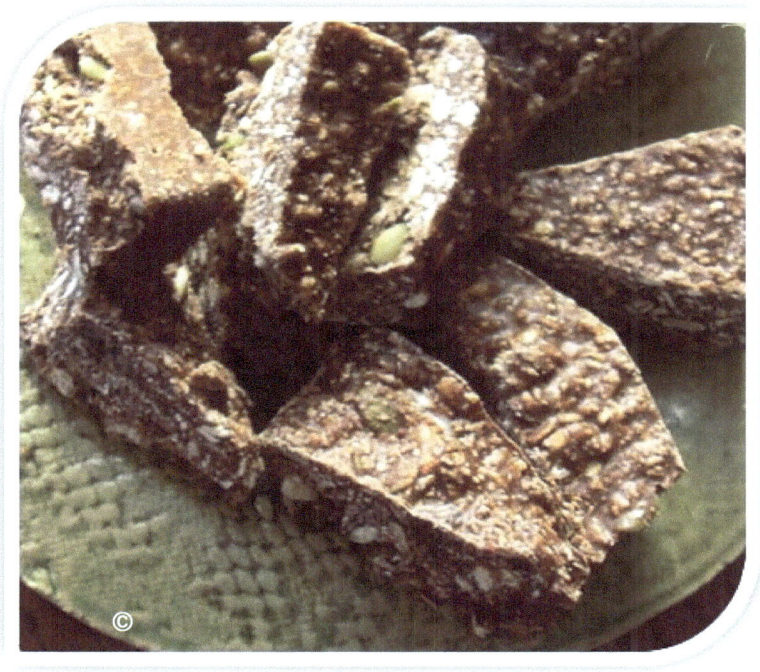

If possible, use either a stainless steel or glass pot & organic ingredients.

Mix liquid

1 ¼ cup virgin coconut oil

¼- cup unpasteurized honey (or to taste)

On the lowest heat - bring honey and coconut oil to a liquid form (coconut oil will liquefy quickly on low heat)

Mix dry ingredients
- 1 cup almonds – freshly ground
- 1 cup sunflower seeds
- 1 cup pumpkin seeds
- 1 cup shredded coconut
- 1 cup carob powder or cocoa powder
- 1 cup rolled oats – (opional - increase almond flour if not using oats)
- 2 handfuls raisins
- ½ tsp. Sea salt

Process
1. Mix liquid and dry ingredients
2. The consistency should be like cookie dough.
3. Press to ¼-½ inch depth in glass or stainless steel pan.
4. Score (even if the score seems to disappear)
5. Place in the freezer for ½-1 hour. If solid, break up into pieces.
6. Store in a zip-lock bag in the fridge or freezer

NOTE: substitute nuts and seeds as desired. Sometimes I substitute walnuts or pecans and sesame seeds.

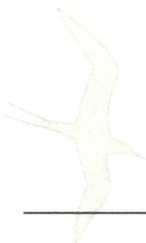

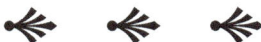

≪ ≪ ≪

NOTES

_____
_____
_____
_____
_____

2. Quick & Easy Apple/Blueberry Pancakes

Wheat free

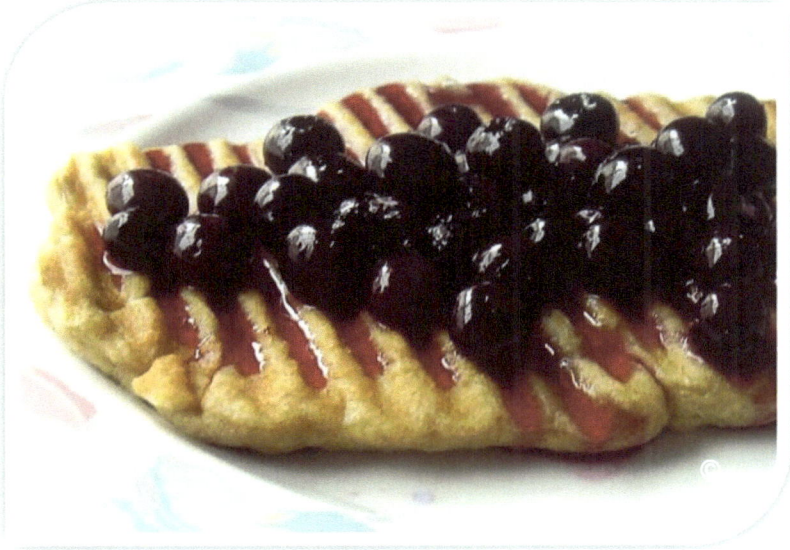

I used an electric sandwich maker to cook these pancakes. If you do not own one, a regular frying pan is all you need. Put a little virgin coconut oil in the pan and heat until it sizzles when you put a drop of water into the pan.

Pour the pancake mix into the pan. If using a frying pan, flip once; lightly brown both sides.

Ingredients
    1 cup light rye or spelt flour (or substitute flour as desired)
    1 tsp. baking powder
       sprinkle of sea salt

1 small organic apple, diced into small pieces
1 egg
½ tbsp extra virgin olive oil
¾ cup liquid (or water, almond milk or goat's milk, etc.)

Process
1. Plug in your electric sandwich maker
2. Mix flour, baking powder, and sea salt
3. In a separate small bowl mix with a fork - egg, oil and liquid.
4. Add the apple pieces to the liquid
5. Add flour mixture to the liquid – mix
6. Drop ½ pancake mixture onto the hot sandwich maker grill or fry pan until golden brown on both sides.
7. Top with Blueberry Topping

Blueberry Topping

Ingredients
1 cup fresh or almost thawed frozen blueberries
2-3 tbsp unpasteurized honey
1 tbsp virgin coconut oil

Process
1. Warm the coconut oil over low heat until clear
2. Add honey to the warm coconut oil
3. Add to the blueberries and stir
4. Pour Blueberry Topping over hot Apple/Blueberry Pancakes

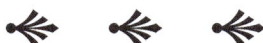

❦ ❦ ❦

3. Tuna & non-GMO Corn on Rye Crisp

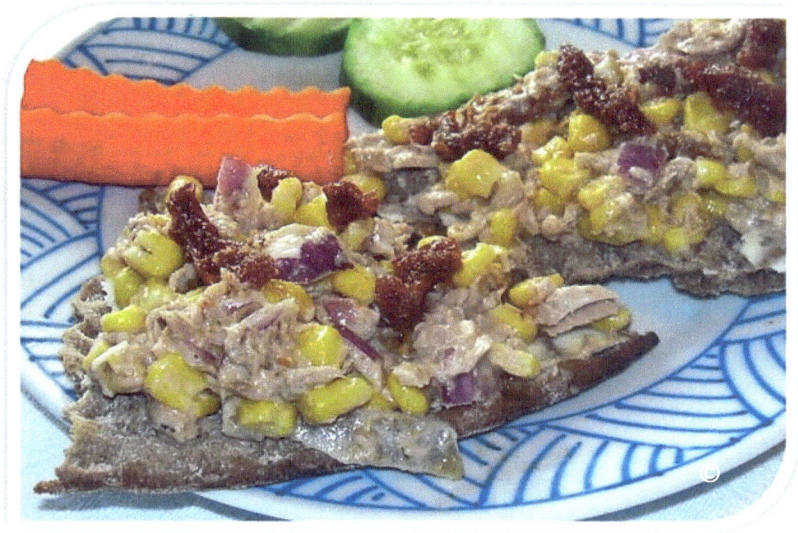

Mix the following

¾ cup cooked non-GMO corn (cold

1 can tuna

2 tbsp chopped red onion

1 tbsp sun dried tomatoes in olive oil

sea salt to taste

In a separate small bowl, mix

1 tbsp mayonnaise (I use Hain Pure Foods Safflower Mayonnaise)

2 tsp extra virgin olive oil

juice of ¼ lemon

1 tsp Apple Cider Vinegar

¼ tsp garlic powder

pepper if desired

Mix the tuna blend and dressing blend together and...

1. Butter the 100% Rye Crisp first if you like
2. Spread the tuna blend onto your Rye Crisp crackers (or crackers of your choice)
3. Top with a few sun-dried tomatoes
4. Serve with carrots sticks and cucumber slices.
5. Serves two.

❦ ❦ ❦

NOTES

_____

_____

_____

_____

_____

_____

_____

_____

_____

_____

_____

_____

_____

_____

_____

_____

_____

_____

4. Stuffed Brown Mushrooms

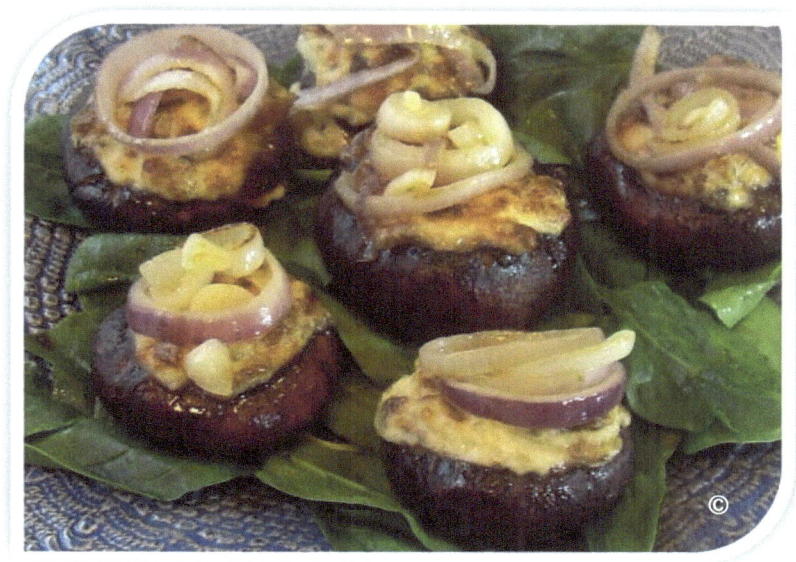

Ingredients

6 big brown mushrooms 2 inches across
3 tbsp grated goat's cheese (or parmesan cheese)
2 finely chopped garlic cloves
1 small red onion cut into 1/4 inch-thick rounds
½ cup mayonnaise (I use Avacado Mayonnaise - Costco)
2 tbsp extra virgin olive oil
1 tsp Bragg Aminos (I use Coconut Secret - Coconut Aminos)
fresh spinach leaves
sea salt

Process

1. Clean mushrooms and remove stems. Set stems aside
2. Place 1 tbsp olive oil and Bragg Aminos into a saucer and mix

3. Dip mushroom tops into the oil mixture letting it soak into the mushroom
4. Lightly sprinkle each cap with sea salt and place onto a plate. Set aside
5. Cut mushroom *stems only* into little pieces
6. Sauté mushroom *stems*, onion rings, garlic in 1 tbsp olive oil
7. Put mayonnaise and parmesan cheese into a mixing bowel
8. Add mushroom onion mix to mayonnaise mix
9. Fill each mushroom with mayonnaise filling
10. Place filled mushrooms into a baking pan.
11. Broil on low for 4 minutes. Broil on high for 2 more minutes.
12. Turn oven heat to 350° F and bake for 3-4 more minutes.
13. Place a handful of fresh spinach onto a serving plate.
14. Place stuffed mushrooms onto spinach bed and serve.

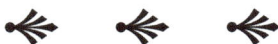

NOTES

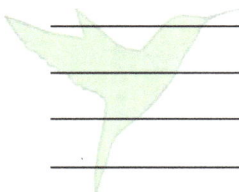

_____
_____
_____
_____
_____
_____
_____
_____

5. Chicken Noodle Turmeric Soup

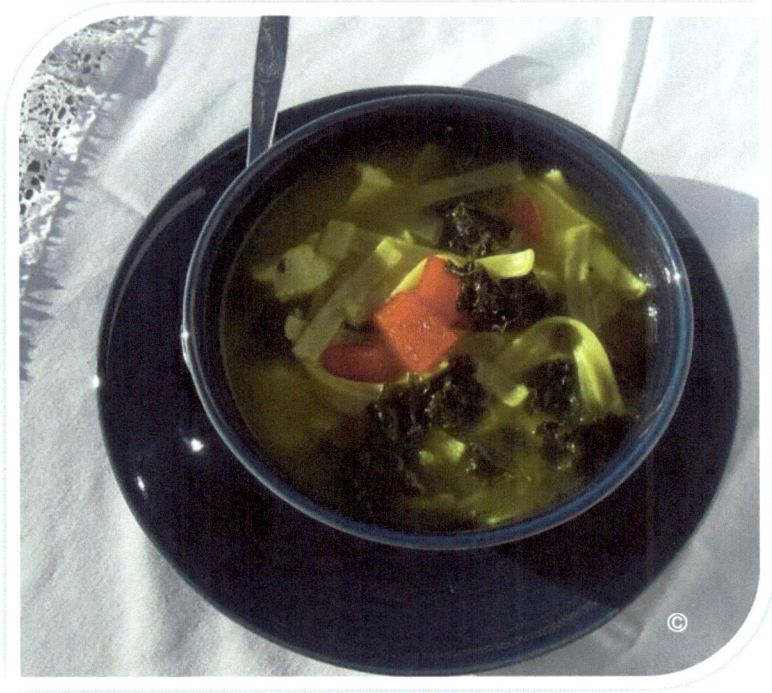

NOTE: Adjust turmeric & hot peppers for taste

Ingredients

    2 quarts of pure water into stainless steel pot
    Brown rice broad noodles (or spelt/egg broad noodles)
    2 cups fresh kale pulled into small pieces (no stems)
    1 medium red pepper cut into pieces
    ½ onion diced
    2 tbsp. olive oil
    1 cube no-MSG organic chicken bouillon cube
    2 bay leaves

1 cup organic chicken breast cut into cubes
1 tsp celery powder
1 tsp. coriander powder
1 tsp. turmeric powder
pinch of hot pepper seeds
sea salt to taste

Process

1. Bring water to a boil
2. Add chopped onion, broad noodles, & 2 tbsp. Olive oil
3. Cook for about 5 minutes
4. Add chopped chicken cubes, kale, and spices
5. Add organic, no-MSG chicken broth cube
6. Cook for another 10 minutes
7. Add red peppers
8. Slow cook for a few more minutes until cooked.
9. Serve

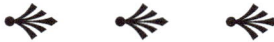

NOTES

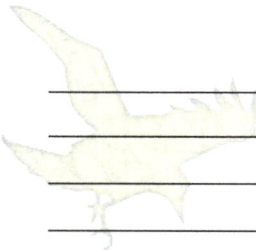

6. Beet Borscht

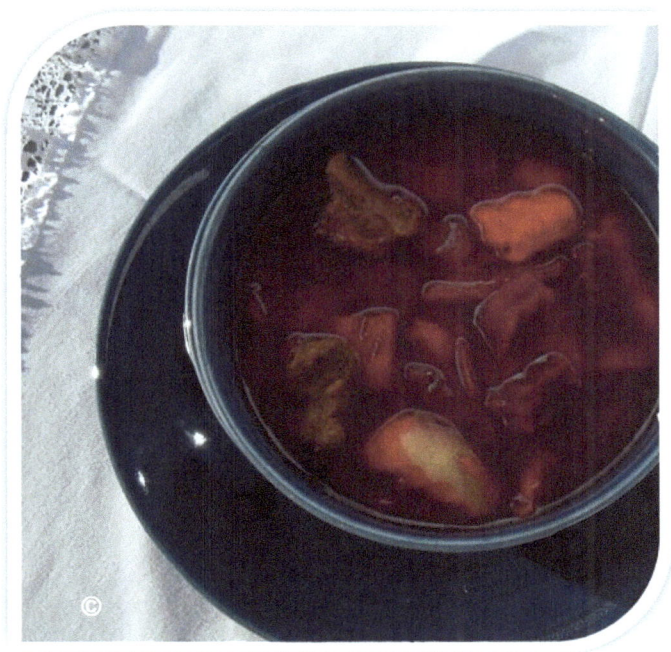

Ingredients

2 quarts water

1 ½ cup rinsed and lightly seared organic stewing beef - cut into small pieces

1 medium onion diced

1 tbsp butter

2 medium red beets cut into cubes

1 large carrot diced

2 potatoes cut into cubes

1 colored pepper cut into thin strips

2 bay leaves

2 cups red cabbage cut into thin strips

1 large tomato blended (or can of crushed tomatoes)

8 peppercorns
2 tsp. dried dill or more if you are using fresh dill
2 tbsp miso (or no-MSG organic beef or vegetable bouillon)
sea salt

Process

1. Bring water to a boil
2. Add stewing beef and bay leaves
3. Continue to cook on med. to low heat
4. Sauté onions in butter
5. Add sautéed onions to broth
6. Let simmer for 1 hour or until meat is tender
7. Then add vegetables, dill, and peppercorns
8. Continue to cook on medium heat until all the vegetables are tender
9. Add miso (or no-MSG organic beef or vegetable bouillon cube)
10. Sea salt to taste
11. Serve as is or with a tbsp of sour cream or yogurt

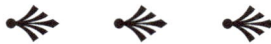

NOTES

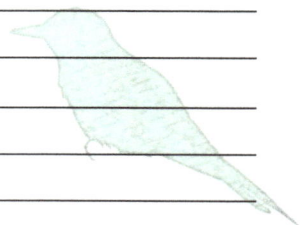

7. Potato Carrot Chicken Soup

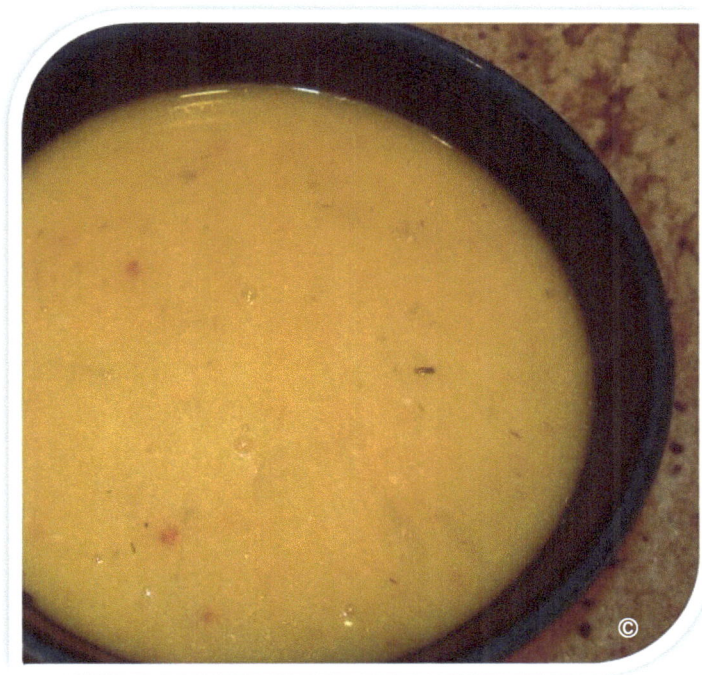

This is an excellent soup to make out of leftover mashed potatoes, carrots and chicken dinner

Ingredients
2 quarts of water
½ onion diced and lightly sautéed
2 cups cooked mashed potato
4 large carrots, cooked and blended
2 tbsp Miso or 1 cube no-MSG chicken bouillon cube
½ tsp dried or fresh dill
1 tsp. dried or fresh chopped rosemary
1 tsp garlic powder or 2 cloves fresh garlic minced
½ tsp celery powder

¼ tsp hot pepper seeds
1 cup cooked chicken cut into small cubes
3 tbsp brown rice flour
½ cup yogurt
½ cup goat's milk or substitute milk of your choice
sea salt to taste

Process

1. Use a stainless steel pot and bring water to a boil
2. Add onion, potatoes, carrots, chicken, miso and spices
3. Bring to a boil.
4. Add chopped chicken, kale
5. Add chicken broth bouillon cube
6. Bring to a light boil
7. Blend brown rice flour into yogurt and milk
8. Add to soup mixture - stir frequently
9. Cook for a few minutes until thickened
10. Add sea salt to taste
11. Serve with sour dough rye bread

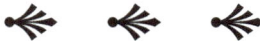

NOTES

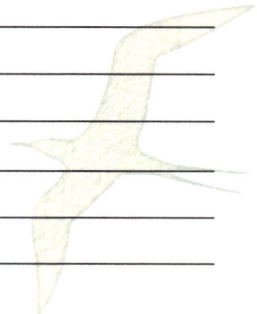

8. Sweet Potato & Tomato Soup

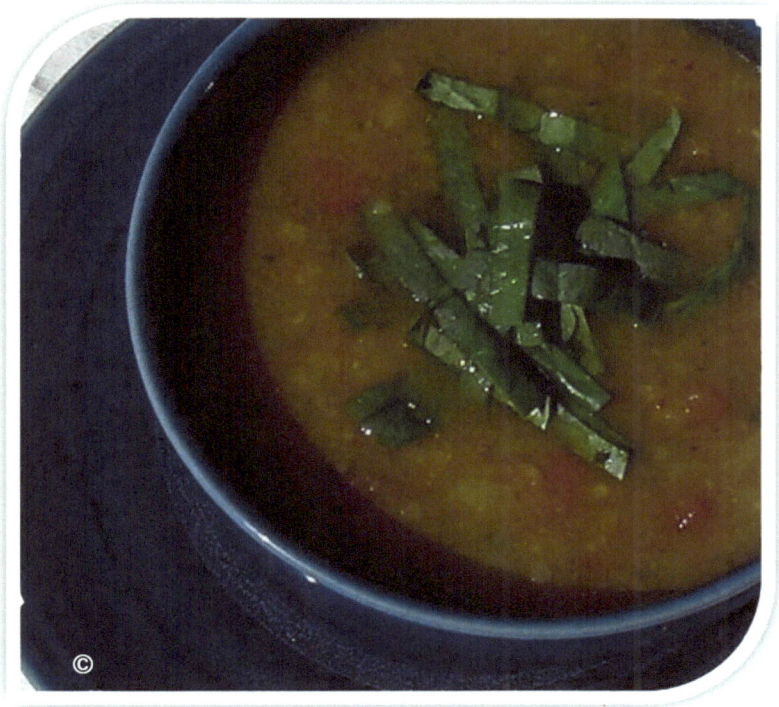

Ingredients
Dice **the follow vegetables into small pieces:**
6 medium tomatoes
1 small cucumber or zucchini
1 small onion
1 red pepper
2 garlic cloves
Mix and set aside

Process
1. Cut 2 medium sweet potatoes into small pieces
2. Cook until soft
3. Mash or blend until creamy
4. Put 4 cups filtered water into a stainless steel pot
5. Bring to a boil
6. **Add**

   diced vegetables

   mashed sweet potatoes

   2 tbsp miso (or no-msg organic vegetable bouillon cube)

   1 tsp. Italian herb mix

   1 tsp. celery powder

   1 tsp. turmeric powder

   1 tbsp virgin olive oil

   sea salt
7. Cook on medium heat for 10 minutes
8. Top with 5-6 baby spinach leaves cut diagonally

Serves 4 people

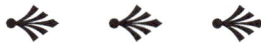

❮❮ ❮❮ ❮❮

NOTES

_____

_____

_____

_____

_____

_____

_____

9. Quick & Easy Vegetable Pea Soup

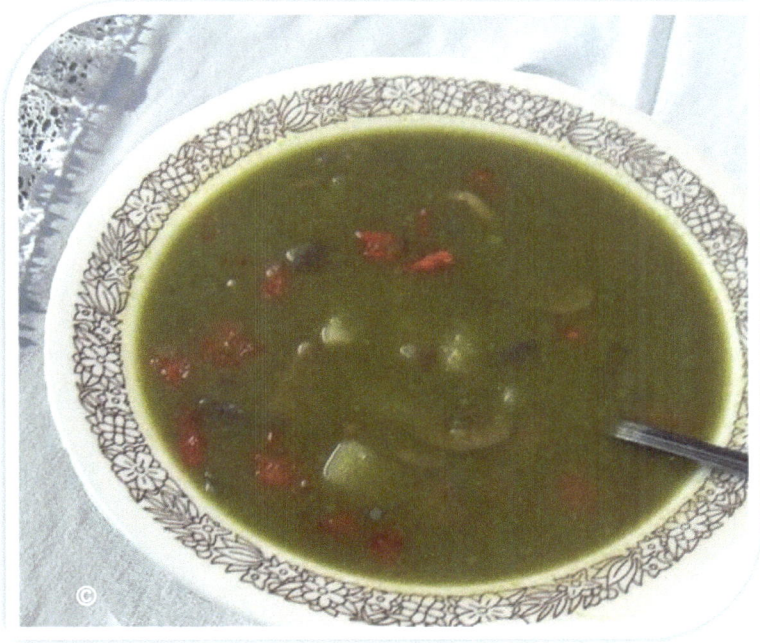

Ingredients

4½ cups water
1 large potato
1 large carrot
1 small onion diced
4 - 6 sliced fresh mushrooms
2 cups frozen peas
2 tbsp non-GMO liquid Bragg Aminos
2 tsp paprika
1 tbsp extra virgin olive oil
2 tbsp flour (I use spelt, tapioca or brown rice flour)
Sea salt

Process

1. Dice onion, potato, and carrot
2. Sauté onions & mushrooms in extra-virgin olive oil and 1 tsp Bragg.
3. Set aside
4. Blend thawed peas and 1 cup of water
5. Put 3 cups water into a stainless steel pot
6. Add blended peas
7. Add diced potato, carrot, and sautéed onion and mushrooms
8. Add remaining Bragg Aminos and paprika
9. Bring to a light boil, stirring often
10. Let soup cook on low to medium heat for 20 minutes. Stir ever so often.
11. In remaining ½ cup water, mix flour until smooth
12. Slowly pour flour mixture into soup, stirring constantly
13. Cook on med or low heat for another 10 minutes
14. Sprinkle with sea salt as desired

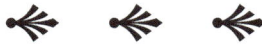

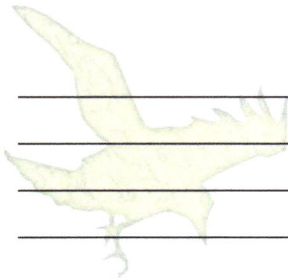

NOTES

_____

_____

_____

_____

_____

_____

_____

_____

_____

10. Green Bean Vegetable Soup

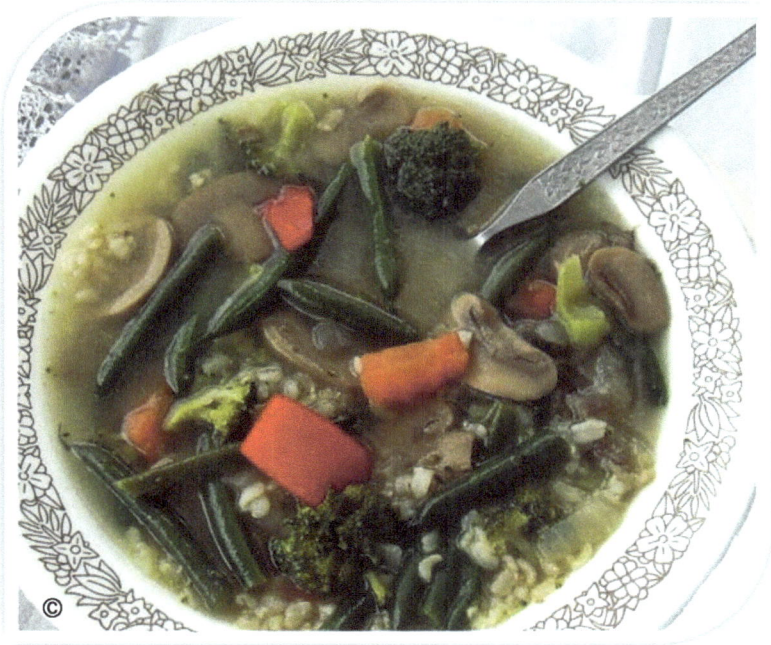

Ingredients

4 cups pure water

1 ½ cup fresh green beans cut in half

1 cup broccoli flowers

1 red pepper cut into pieces

1 small onion chopped

6 - 8 small mushrooms sliced

1 small carrot cut into small pieces or slices

1 cube no-MSG organic vegetable bouillon cube

2 bay leaves

6 pepper corns

½ tsp. powdered garlic (optional)

½ cup cooked brown rice
1 tsp. fresh or dried dill
sea salt

Process
1. Put water into a stainless steel pot and bring to a boil
2. Sauté mushrooms and onions in a small amount of extra virgin olive oil
3. Set aside
4. Add the following to the boiling water
   green beans
   red pepper
   sautéed onions and mushrooms
   carrot pieces
   bay leaves
   pepper corns
   garlic powder

NOTE: use ½ cup hot water to dissolve bouillon cube - once dissolved - pour into pot of hot water

5. Cook over medium heat until beans are partially cooked and still bright green
6. Add
   broccoli
   cooked brown rice
   garlic powder
   dill
   sea salt to taste
7. Cook for a few more minutes until beans and broccoli are tender but still bright green. Do not over-cook!

❰ ❰ ❰

11. Pork Broth Vegetable Soup

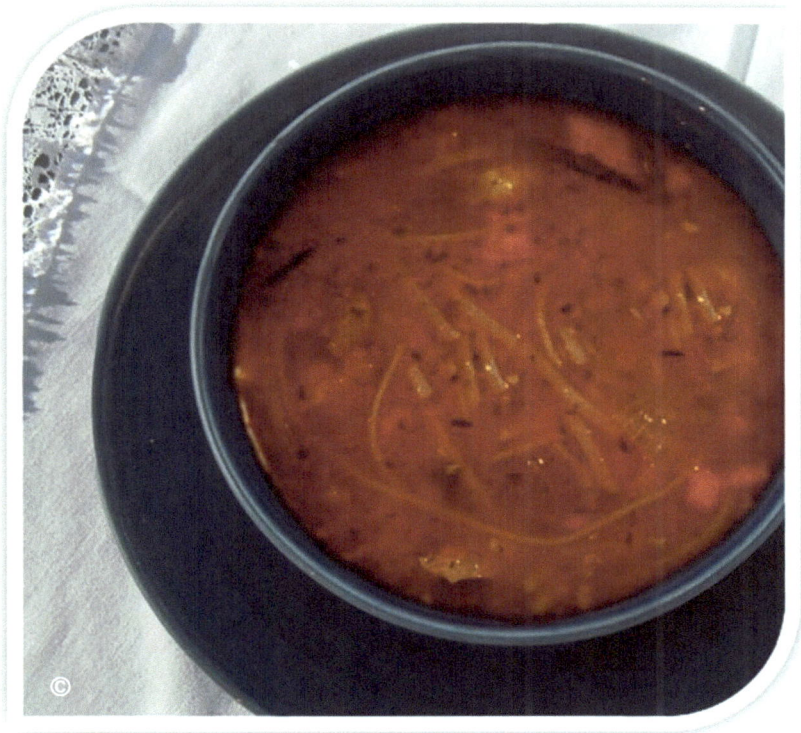

Visit Dr. Josh Axe's website to learn more about bone broth, and why you want to incorporate it into your diet.

https://draxe.com/the-healing-power-of-bone-broth-for-digestion-arthritis-and-cellulite/

You can use **organic** chicken, lamb, beef bones as well. *"...bone broth is rich in minerals that support the immune system and contains healing compounds like collagen, glutamine, glycine and proline. The collagen in bone broth heals your gut lining and reduces intestinal inflammation."*

Day 1

1. Bring 4 cups filtered water to boil
2. Add organic pork bones (can use leftover bones from pork ribs)
3. Add 2 tbsp. apple cider vinegar (helps to pull the minerals out of bones)
4. Bring to a boil and simmer bones for 24 hours.
5. Remove bones - check for small bone pieces.
6. Cool and put in the fridge to be used the following day.

Day 2

1. Remove the solidified fat from broth, discard and bring broth to a boil.
2. Dice the following vegetables into small pieces
   1 carrot   1 small onion
   1 red pepper   2 garlic cloves
   3 fresh tomatoes
3. Puree the diced vegetables
4. Add to above ingredients to the broth
5. Dissolve 1 organic veg. bouillon cube in 1 cup hot water
6. Add to broth and stir
7. Add
   1 tsp. rosemary - fresh or dried
   ½ tsp. thyme -fresh or dried
   1 tsp. dill - fresh or dried
   2 tsp. paprika powder
   squirt of mustard
   2 tsp organic molasses
   sea salt to taste
   1 cup brown rice noodles
8. Cook over medium heat until noodles are done. Stir every so often.

12. Stuffed Sweet Colored Peppers

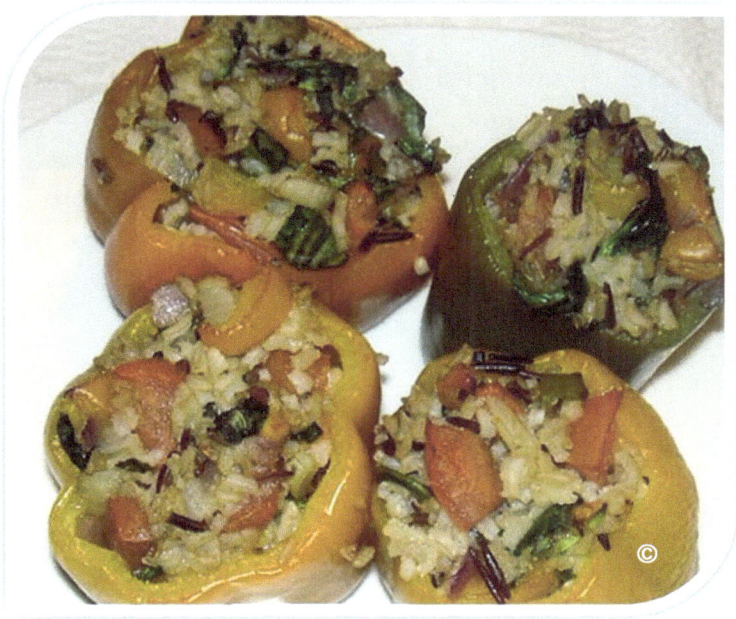

Ingredients

4 whole large, colored peppers
1 stalk diced celery
½ cup diced colored peppers
¼ cup chopped onion
2 cups cooked brown rice
1 chopped tomato
1 handful of fresh spinach chopped
1 tsp honey
½ tsp sea salt
1 tsp garlic powder
¼ tsp sweet basil
¼ tsp oregano
2 tbsp liquid non-GMO Bragg soya sauce

Process

1. Cut the tops off the peppers and remove centers.
2. Steam the peppers in a small amount of water - about 8 minutes.
3. Lightly simmer celery, diced peppers, and onion in a small amount of water.
4. Drain celery, peppers, and onion - add honey, sea salt, garlic powder, basil and oregano - mix
5. Add chopped spinach and chopped tomato – mix
6. Add mixture to cooked brown rice - mix
7. Stuff steamed peppers with rice mixture.
8. Put a little water in the bottom of a glass or stainless steel baking dish (about ¼" deep)
9. Place stuffed peppers into the pan
10. Bake at 350° F for 30 minutes.

NOTES

13. Sprouted Gluten-Free Bread Pudding

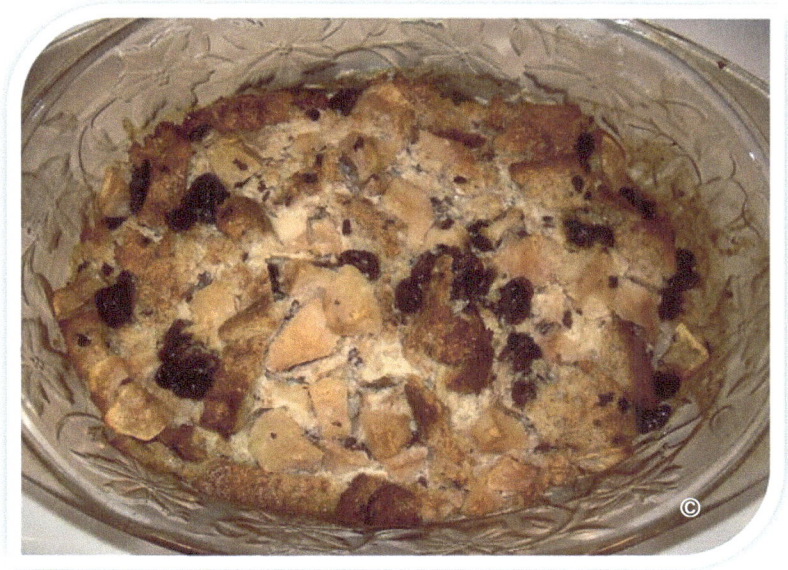

Ingredients

Organic sprouted gluten-free bread cut into small cubes
½ cup raisins
1 large organic apple diced.
2 ½ cups almond or goat's milk
3 tbsp. mini tapioca
4 eggs
sea salt
2 tsp. cinnamon
¼ cup real maple syrup

Process

1. Mix **and set aside**
   bread cubes
   raisins
   organic apple diced

2. Beat eggs and ½ cup milk till frothy
3. In a sauce pan combine

      2 cups almond milk or goat's milk

      3 tbsp. mini tapioca

      a pinch of sea salt

      2 tsp cinnamon

4. Add the frothy egg and milk mixture and stir
5. Cook liquid over medium heat stirring constantly, until it begins to thicken
6. Pour liquid over set aside bread, raisins, and apple
7. Mix until bread is soaked
8. Spread a few drops of oil on the bottom & sides of baking dish
9. Scrape bread pudding into the baking dish
10. Bake at 350° F for approximately 1 hour
11. Remove from oven
12. Evenly pour ¼ cup real maple syrup over the pudding
13. Serve alone or with cream, whipped cream, ice cream or cream substitute i.e. coconut cream

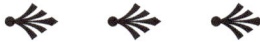

NOTES

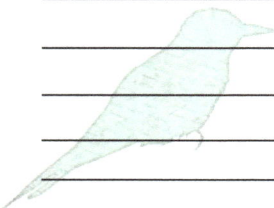

About the Author

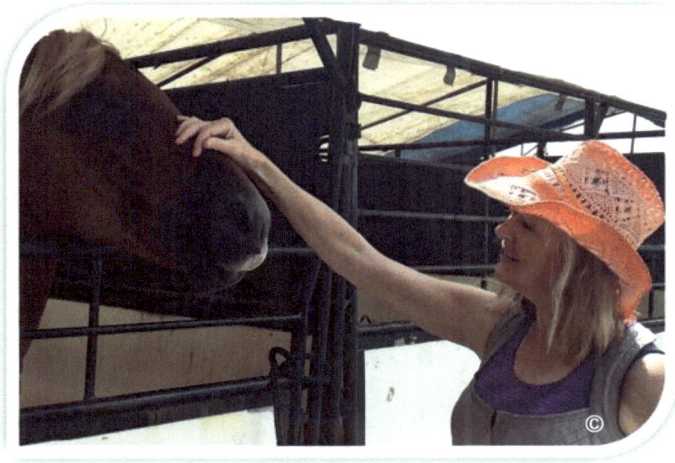

Carrie is an award-winning artist and author. ***Roadlocks to Hell*** was a Kindle best-seller. She writes for adults and children, fantasy and adventure being her favorite styles.

A gifted storyteller, Carrie's works reflect her love of animals, nature, and sometimes, a snowy winter's day. She credits all of her accomplishments to a loving Almighty God. She says, "Having a personal relationship with Jesus Christ of the Bible is the strength of my life."

Carrie has always participated in athletics of various types. She grew up in a small southern Manitoba farming community—barefoot and adventurous.

Carrie is an encourager and facilitator who helps others realize their dreams of publishing their books.

Carrie has a M.Min (Professional Writer) and D.Min (Fine Arts and Media).

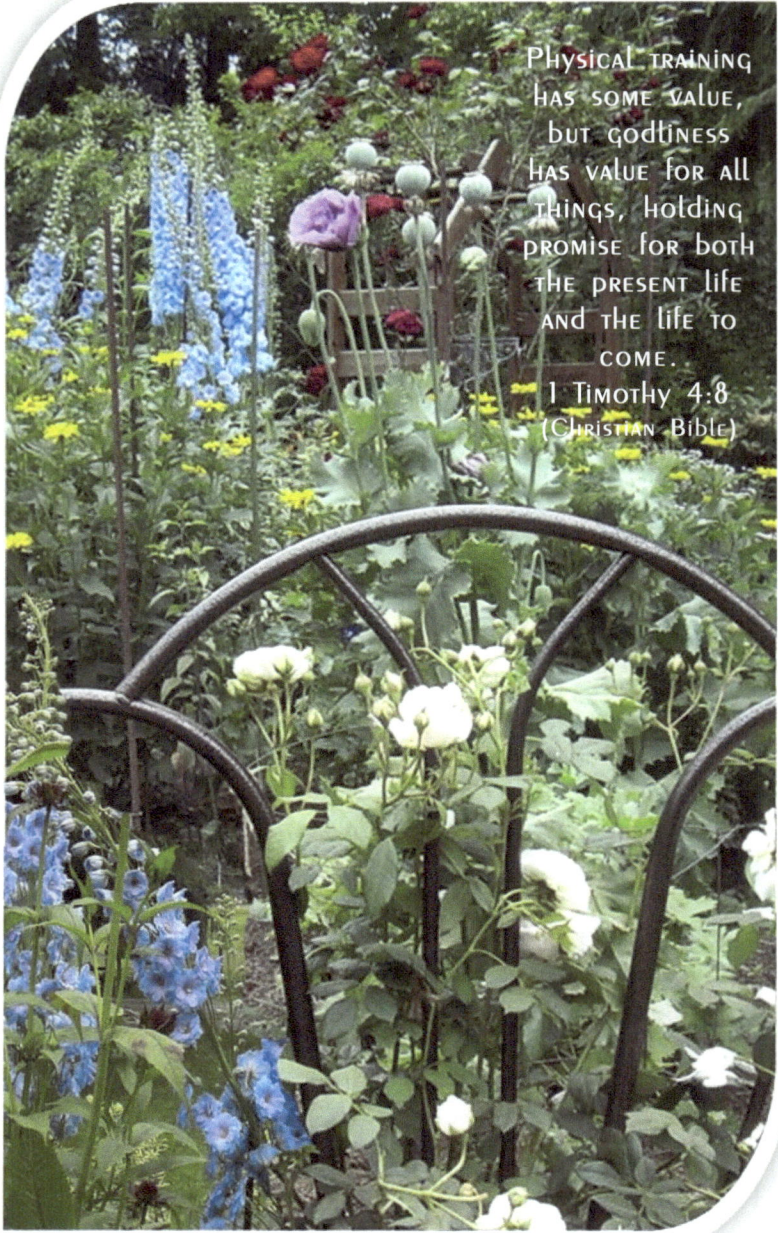

Physical training has some value, but godliness has value for all things, holding promise for both the present life and the life to come.

1 Timothy 4:8
(Christian Bible)

Published works

Books available on **Amazon** here: **http://amzn.to/2piDLGR**
or you can contact the publisher directly

The RYDER - fantasy adventure
http://theryder.wordpress.com

Treasure Trap – sequel to The Ryder - fantasy adventure

Newfies to the Rescue - tales of the Newfoundland Dog

Chuzzle's Incredible Journey - children's book co-authored with
Minde Wachsmann

Roadblocks to Hell - fiction based on a true story - drama-filled, action-
packed story of redemption
http://roadblockstohell.com

Finding Christmas - A Mouse in Search of Christmas

Author's website: **http://www.carriewachsmann.com/blog**

Published by
HeartBeat Productions Inc.
Box 633, Abbotsford, BC, Canada V2T 6Z8
email: info@heartbeat1.com
604.852.3769

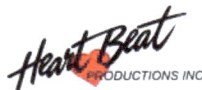

www.ingramcontent.com/pod-product-compliance
Lightning Source LLC
Chambersburg PA
CBHW041214270326
41930CB00001B/11